MCQs in Clinical Pathology

A J Bint MB ChB, FRCPath

Consultant Microbiologist,
The Royal Victoria Infirmary, Newcastle-upon-Tyne

A D Burt MD (Hons), BSc (Hons), MB ChB, MRCPath

Postgraduate Sub-Dean of Medicine & Senior Lecturer in Pathology, University of
Newcastle-upon-Tyne and Honorary Consultant Histopathologist,
The Royal Victoria Infirmary, Newcastle-upon-Tyne

M F Laker MD, Dip Biochem, FRCPath

Reader in Clinical Biochemistry and Metabolic Medicine, University of Newcastle-
upon-Tyne, and Consultant in Clinical Biochemistry,
The Royal Victoria Infirmary, Newcastle-upon-Tyne

M M Reid MD, BSc, FRCP, MRCPath, DCH

Honorary Senior Lecturer, Departments of Medicine and Child Health, University of
Newcastle-upon-Tyne, and Consultant Haematologist,
The Royal Victoria Infirmary, Newcastle-upon-Tyne

W B SAUNDERS COMPANY LIMITED
London   Philadelphia   Toronto   Sydney   Tokyo

W. B. Saunders Company Ltd 24–28 Oval Road
London NW1 7DX

The Curtis Center
Independence Square West
Philadelphia, PA 19106-3399, USA

Harcourt Brace & Company
55 Horner Avenue
Toronto, Ontario M8Z 4X6,
Canada

Harcourt Brace & Company,
   Australia
30–52 Smidmore Street
Marrickville, NSW 2204, Australia

Harcourt Brace & Company, Japan
Ichibancho Central Building,
22–1 Ichibancho
Chiyoda-ku, Tokyo 102, Japan

A catalogue record for this book is available from the British
Library

ISBN 0-7020-1782-5

Typeset by Selwood Systems, Midsomer Norton
Printed and bound in Great Britain by
WBC Book Manufacturers, Bridgend

Contents

Preface

Clinical pathology is the scientific foundation of modern medical practice, and therefore forms a fundamental knowledge base for the whole of medicine. This book of multiple-choice questions (MCQs) has therefore been produced as an aid to all those studying for examinations in the pathological sciences. It should be useful not only for undergraduate medical students but also for postgraduates working for examinations for membership of UK Royal Colleges, or equivalent postgraduate qualifications.

The questions are grouped in four main specialties: Medical Microbiology (including virology), Histopathology, Clinical Biochemistry, and Haematology (including some immunology). The first part of the book comprises the questions, and the second part the answers with short explanatory comments. The standard of the questions is aimed at undergraduate level, but about 5% of the questions would be considered as difficult by this group. Many of the questions are distinctly clinically orientated.

MCQs are now common to most undergraduate and postgraduate examinations. It is crucial that students are familiar with this type of question, and adopt a strategy for answering them. All of the questions in this book have the same structure: a statement (or stem) followed by five completions (or items). The completions may be true or false. The best strategy for answering this type of question depends to some extent on the scoring system, but we would always discourage too much guessing. We suggest that readers try to answer at least 10 to 20 questions before looking up the answers. For those who attempt all of the questions, it will do no harm to have another go. Good luck!

QUESTIONS

Medical Microbiology – Questions

1. Compared to Gram-negative bacteria, Gram-positive bacteria:

  A. have cell walls containing more peptidoglycan.
  B. are less sensitive to penicillin.
  C. are more resistant to lysozyme.
  D. include some spore-forming species.
  E. may produce endotoxin.

  A. . . . . .   B. . . . . .   C. . . . . .   D. . . . . .   E. . . . . .

2. Viruses:

  A. are 1–3 μm in size.
  B. can reproduce only within host cells.
  C. contain ribosomes.
  D. have a cell wall.
  E. may carry genetic information on DNA or RNA.

  A. . . . . .   B. . . . . .   C. . . . . .   D. . . . . .   E. . . . . .

3. *Staphylococcus aureus:*

  A. is a Gram-positive coccus.
  B. forms long chains.
  C. is coagulase positive.
  D. can cause food poisoning.
  E. is motile by means of a polar flagellum.

  A. . . . . .   B. . . . . .   C. . . . . .   D. . . . . .   E. . . . . .

4. Bacterial exotoxins:

    A.   are usually found in Gram-positive bacteria.
    B.   can be converted to toxoids.
    C.   are high-molecular weight proteins.
    D.   are heat stable.
    E.   contain lipopolysaccharide.

        A. . . . . .   B. . . . . .   C. . . . . .   D. . . . . .   E. . . . . .

5. Plasmids:

    A.   are extrachromosomal pieces of DNA.
    B.   can carry antibiotic-resistance genes.
    C.   replicate autonomously.
    D.   can be transferred between bacteria.
    E.   possess flagella.

        A. . . . . .   B. . . . . .   C. . . . . .   D. . . . . .   E. . . . . .

6. *Clostridium perfringens*:

    A.   is a Gram-positive coccus.
    B.   is a facultative anaerobe.
    C.   produces spores.
    D.   causes gas gangrene.
    E.   causes food poisoning.

        A. . . . . .   B. . . . . .   C. . . . . .   D. . . . . .   E. . . . . .

7. The following are causes of food poisoning:

    A.   *Bacillus cereus.*
    B.   *Bacillus subtilis.*
    C.   *Vibrio parahaemolyticus.*
    D.   *Shigella sonnei.*
    E.   *Clostridium difficile.*

        A. . . . . .   B. . . . . .   C. . . . . .   D. . . . . .   E. . . . . .

8. Ampicillin:

   A. kills bacteria by causing damage to their cell walls.
   B. blocks folic acid reductase.
   C. is destroyed by staphylococcal β-lactamase.
   D. usually inhibits the bactericidal action of other antibiotics.
   E. is stable to the common type of β-lactamase (TEM) found in *Escherichia coli.*

   A. . . . . .   B. . . . . .   C. . . . . .   D. . . . . .   E. . . . . .

9. *Streptococcus pyogenes:*

   A. is α-haemolytic.
   B. is a common bacterial cause of tonsillitis.
   C. can be found in the heart valves of patients with rheumatic fever.
   D. is often resistant to penicillin.
   E. is Gram-positive.

   A. . . . . .   B. . . . . .   C. . . . . .   D. . . . . .   E. . . . . .

10. The following antibiotics work by inhibiting protein synthesis in bacteria:

   A. gentamicin.
   B. penicillin.
   C. erythromycin.
   D. chloramphenicol.
   E. ciprofloxacin.

   A. . . . . .   B. . . . . .   C. . . . . .   D. . . . . .   E. . . . . .

11. The following proteins may be found in the core of a virus:

   A. neuraminidase.
   B. RNA polymerase.
   C. DNA polymerase.
   D. haemagglutinin.
   E. reverse transcriptase.

   A. . . . . .   B. . . . . .   C. . . . . .   D. . . . . .   E. . . . . .

12. Endotoxin:

    A. is found in Gram-positive bacteria.
    B. is a component of lipopolysaccharide.
    C. causes food poisoning.
    D. causes septic shock.
    E. causes macrophages to release endogenous pyrogens.

    A. . . . . B. . . . . C. . . . . D. . . . . E. . . . .

13. The following agents can be used to achieve sterility:

    A. hypochlorite.
    B. ethylene oxide gas.
    C. autoclaving.
    D. dry heat.
    E. ethyl alcohol.

    A. . . . . B. . . . . C. . . . . D. . . . . E. . . . .

14. The following antibiotics inhibit bacterial cell wall synthesis:

    A. vancomycin.
    B. penicillin.
    C. trimethoprim.
    D. bacitracin.
    E. cefuroxime.

    A. . . . . B. . . . . C. . . . . D. . . . . E. . . . .

15. Respiratory syncytial virus (RSV):

    A. is the major cause of viral meningitis in children.
    B. has a genome of double-stranded DNA.
    C. is an enveloped, pleomorphic virus.
    D. is a member of a genus called coronavirus.
    E. causes bronchiolitis in infants.

    A. . . . . B. . . . . C. . . . . D. . . . . E. . . . .

16. The Mantoux test:

 A. is a test for tuberculin hypersensitivity.
 B. involves injecting PPD (purified protein derivative) intramuscularly.
 C. is positive in someone with active tuberculosis.
 D. becomes positive within two weeks of infection.
 E. is more reliable than the Tine test.

 A. . . . . .   B. . . . . .   C. . . . . .   D. . . . . .   E. . . . . .

17. *Pseudomonas aeruginosa*:

 A. is a Gram-positive bacillus.
 B. is a common pathogen in cystic fibrosis patients.
 C. produces a green pigment in culture media.
 D. is usually sensitive to amoxycillin.
 E. is an important cause of infection in burns.

 A. . . . . .   B. . . . . .   C. . . . . .   D. . . . . .   E. . . . . .

18. Recognized causes of community-acquired pneumonia include:

 A. *Chlamydia psittaci.*
 B. *Chlamydia pneumoniae.*
 C. *Proteus mirabilis.*
 D. *Streptococcus pneumoniae.*
 E. *Mycoplasma hominis.*

 A. . . . . .   B. . . . . .   C. . . . . .   D. . . . . .   E. . . . . .

19. Recognized causes of acute, uncomplicated cystitis include:

 A. *Candida albicans.*
 B. *Staphylococcus saprophyticus.*
 C. *Escherichia coli.*
 D. *Pseudomonas aeruginosa.*
 E. *Staphylococcus aureus.*

 A. . . . . .   B. . . . . .   C. . . . . .   D. . . . . .   E. . . . . .

20. In infective endocarditis in patients with no prior heart surgery:

    A. blood cultures are rarely positive.
    B. the mortality rate is <5%.
    C. viridans streptococci are the most common cause.
    D. flucloxacillin is appropriate blind starting therapy.
    E. fever is found in 80% of cases.

      A. . . . . .   B. . . . . .   C. . . . . .   D. . . . . .   E. . . . . .

21. *Streptococcus pneumoniae*:

    A. is a Gram-positive diplococcus.
    B. produces β-haemolysis on blood agar.
    C. is motile.
    D. is sensitive to optochin.
    E. has a polysaccharide capsule as a virulence factor.

      A. . . . . .   B. . . . . .   C. . . . . .   D. . . . . .   E. . . . . .

22. Pseudomembranous colitis:

    A. is caused by *Clostridium perfringens.*
    B. is unrelated to previous antibiotic therapy.
    C. diagnosis is aided by detection of toxin in faeces.
    D. can be treated appropriately with oral vancomycin.
    E. causes diarrhoea.

      A. . . . . .   B. . . . . .   C. . . . . .   D. . . . . .   E. . . . . .

23. Recognized causes of acute meningitis in primary school children include:

    A. *Streptococcus pneumoniae.*
    B. group B β-haemolytic streptococcus.
    C. *Haemophilus influenzae.*
    D. *Neisseria meningitidis.*
    E. *Streptococcus pyogenes.*

      A. . . . . .   B. . . . . .   C. . . . . .   D. . . . . .   E. . . . . .

24. In typhoid fever:

    A.   diarrhoea is a principal symptom in the first week of illness.
    B.   blood cultures are typically positive in the first week.
    C.   the incubation period is usually less than 7 days.
    D.   *Salmonella typhi* localizes in Peyer's patches.
    E.   *Salmonella typhi* can be found in farm animals.

    A. . . . . .   B. . . . . .   C. . . . . .   D. . . . . .   E. . . . . .

25. The following statements are correct:

    A.   legionnaires' disease is a recognized type of community-acquired pneumonia.
    B.   person-to-person spread is an important mechanism of transmission of *Legionella*.
    C.   *Legionella pneumophila* is widely distributed in aqueous environments.
    D.   *Legionella pneumophila* is fastidious in its growth requirements in the laboratory.
    E.   erythromycin is an appropriate antibiotic for legionnaires' disease.

    A. . . . . .   B. . . . . .   C. . . . . .   D. . . . . .   E. . . . . .

26. The following microorganisms are correctly paired with their usual mode of transmission:

    A.   *Mycobacterium tuberculosis* – droplet nuclei.
    B.   *Giardia lamblia* – direct contact.
    C.   *Salmonella typhimurium* – food.
    D.   HIV – aerosol.
    E.   *leptospira icterohaemorrhagiae* – water.

    A. . . . . .   B. . . . . .   C. . . . . .   D. . . . . .   E. . . . . .

27. Hepatitis A:

    A.   has an incubation period of 6 weeks to 6 months.
    B.   can produce a carrier state.
    C.   is spread by the faecal–oral route.
    D.   often spreads in epidemics.
    E.   can be found in contaminated shellfish.

    A. . . . . .   B. . . . . .   C. . . . . .   D. . . . . .   E. . . . . .

28. The following organisms are inherently resistant to gentamicin:

A. *Pseudomonas aeruginosa.*
B. *Staphylococcus aureus.*
C. *Proteus mirabilis.*
D. *Bacteroides fragilis.*
E. *Enterococcus faecalis.*

A. . . . . .   B. . . . . .   C. . . . . .   D. . . . . .   E. . . . . .

29. The following antibiotics are regarded as safe to use in the first trimester of pregnancy:

A. cephalexin.
B. trimethoprim.
C. tetracycline.
D. amoxycillin.
E. nitrofurantoin.

A. . . . . .   B. . . . . .   C. . . . . .   D. . . . . .   E. . . . . .

30. Antibiotic prophylaxis can be used to prevent:

A. enteric fever in hospital staff contacts of a case.
B. meningococcal meningitis in family contacts of a case.
C. wound sepsis following cholecystectomy.
D. urinary tract infection in a patient with a long-term urinary catheter.
E. *Pneumocystis carinii* pneumonia in a child with leukaemia.

A. . . . . .   B. . . . . .   C. . . . . .   D. . . . . .   E. . . . . .

31. *Staphylococcus aureus* is a recognized cause of the following diseases:

A. impetigo.
B. scarlet fever.
C. toxic shock syndrome.
D. haemolytic uraemic syndrome.
E. scalded skin syndrome.

A. . . . . .   B. . . . . .   C. . . . . .   D. . . . . .   E. . . . . .

✓ **32.** The following disinfectants are suitable for preoperative skin disinfection:

    A. glutaraldehyde.
    B. ethylene oxide.
    C. phenol.
    D. povidone-iodine.
    E. chlorhexidine.

    A. . . . . .   B. . . . . .   C. . . . . .   D. . . . . .   E. . . . . . .

33. *Haemophilus influenzae:*

    A. is a Gram-negative bacillus.
    B. requires X factor, but not V factor.
    C. type b causes epiglottitis.
    D. produces the satellite phenomenon around staphylococcal colonies.
    E. is a cause of influenza.

    A. . . . . .   B. . . . . .   C. . . . . .   D. . . . . .   E. . . . . . .

✓ **34.** The following statements about bacterial structure and function are correct:

    A. endospores are heat sensitive.
    B. pili are organs of locomotion.
    C. ribosomes carry hereditary information.
    D. peptidoglycan contains *N*-acetylmuramic acid.
    E. porins are involved in nutrient transport.

    A. . . . . .   B. . . . . .   C. . . . . .   D. . . . . .   E. . . . . . .

35. The following statements about malaria are correct:

    A. malaria due to *Plasmodium falciparum* can relapse up to 30 years after the original illness.
    B. primaquine (or a similar drug) is used to prevent relapses of vivax malaria.
    C. antimalarial prophylaxis need to be taken only from one week before travel to the malarious area until one week after leaving the area.
    D. quinine can be used to treat falciparum malaria.
    E. *Plasmodium malariae* has an exo-erythrocytic cycle.

    A. . . . . .   B. . . . . .   C. . . . . .   D. . . . . .   E. . . . . . .

36. Chlamydiae:

    A.   contain peptidoglycan in their cell wall.
    B.   exist in one form: the elementary body.
    C.   cause Q fever.
    D.   cause pelvic inflammatory disease.
    E.   are sensitive to tetracycline.

    A. . . . .   B. . . . . .   C. . . . . .   D. . . . . .   E. . . . . .

37. The following diseases are correctly paired with an insect vector:

    A.   bubonic plague – tick.
    B.   scrub typhus – mite.
    C.   lyme disease – mosquito.
    D.   sleeping sickness – tsetse fly.
    E.   epidemic typhus – flea.

    A. . . . .   B. . . . . .   C. . . . . .   D. . . . . .   E. . . . . .

38. The following bacteria are correctly paired with a toxin:

    A.   *Clostridium perfringens* – endotoxin.
    B.   *Streptococcus pyogenes* – erythrogenic toxin.
    C.   *Neisseria meningitidis* – phospholipase.
    D.   *Escherichia coli* – verotoxin.
    E.   *Bacillus cereus* – enterotoxin.

    A. . . . .   B. . . . . .   C. . . . . .   D. . . . . .   E. . . . . .

39. *Mycobacterium tuberculosis*:

    A.   cells divide every 2–3 hours.
    B.   can be stained by the Ziehl–Neelsen stain.
    C.   colonies produce pigment when exposed to light.
    D.   infection is characterized by granulomas in human tissues.
    E.   can be treated with pyrazinamide.

    A. . . . .   B. . . . . .   C. . . . . .   D. . . . . .   E. . . . . .

✓ **40.** *Candida albicans* is normally sensitive to:

    A. amphotericin B.
    B. fluconazole.
    C. metronidazole.
    D. griseofulvin.
    E. nystatin.

    A. . . . . .   B. . . . . .   C. . . . . .   D. . . . . .   E. . . . . .

41. The following statements about diphtheria are correct:

    A. *Corynebacterium diphtheriae* is an aerobic, Gram-positive rod.
    B. a positive Dick test indicates no immunity.
    C. a selective culture medium for *Corynebacterium diphtheriae* contains selenite.
    D. the genes for toxin production in corynebacteria are carried on a plasmid.
    E. diphtheria vaccine is a live, attenuated vaccine.

    A. . . . . .   B. . . . . .   C. . . . . .   D. . . . . .   E. . . . . .

42. Recognized causes of acute meningitis in neonates include:

    A. *Haemophilus influenzae.*
    B. *Neisseria meningitidis.*
    C. group β-haemolytic streptococcus.
    D. *Listeria monocytogenes.*
    E. *Escherichia coli.*

    A. . . . . .   B. . . . . .   C. . . . . ,.   D. . . . . .   E. . . . . .

43. The following antibiotics are correctly matched with a recognized adverse effect:

    A. benzylpenicillin – epileptiform fits.
    B. gentamicin – aplastic anaemia.
    C. chloramphenicol – vestibular toxicity.
    D. tetracycline – tooth discoloration.
    E. vancomycin – nephrotoxicity.

    A. . . . . .   B. . . . . .   C. . . . . .   D. . . . . .   E. . . . . .

44. The following CSF (cerebrospinal fluid) findings are typical of an acute, bacterial meningitis in an adult:

    A.   500 lymphocytes per mm^3.
    B.   turbid.
    C.   protein 2.0 g/l.
    D.   glucose 3.0 mmol/l (60% of blood level).
    E.   positive for bacterial antigen.

    A. . . . . .   B. . . . . .   C. . . . . .   D. . . . . .   E. . . . . .

45. The following statements about operon functions are correct:

    A.   operons consist of genes and nucleotide sequences.
    B.   the regulator gene codes for the synthesis of a repressor.
    C.   the promotor gene codes for the synthesis of RNA polymerase.
    D.   the operator is a sequence of nucleotides that binds the repressor protein.
    E.   inducible operons are primarily involved in the control of catabolic processes.

    A. . . . . .   B. . . . . .   C. . . . . .   D. . . . . .   E. . . . . .

46. The following statements about tetanus are correct:

    A.   *Clostridium tetani* has terminal spores.
    B.   *Clostridium tetani* is motile.
    C.   tetanospasmin causes flaccid paralysis.
    D.   *Clostridium tetani* gives a positive Nagler test.
    E.   tetanospasmin prevents the release of inhibitory mediators of motor neurones.

    A. . . . . .   B. . . . . .   C. . . . . .   D. . . . . .   E. . . . . .

47. The following statements about syphilis are correct:

    A.   *Treponema pallidum* is motile by means of a polar flagellum.
    B.   gummas are typical of tertiary syphilis.
    C.   the VDRL test detects reagin.
    D.   a hard chancre is typical of secondary syphilis.
    E.   the FTA-ABS (Fluorescent Treponemal Antibody-Absorption) test is sensitive in all stages of syphilis.

    A. . . . . .   B. . . . . .   C. . . . . .   D. . . . . .   E. . . . . .

48. The following statements about bacteriophage are correct:

A. lysogeny is the relationship between the host cell and a lytic phage.
B. the host cell's phenotype may be changed by lysogenic conversion.
C. areas of clearing on lawned agar caused by phage are called foci.
D. *Corynebacterium diphtheriae* is only virulent when it carries a temperate phage.
E. bacterial conjugation is mediated by phage.

A. . . . . .   B. . . . . .   C. . . . . .   D. . . . . .   E. . . . . .

49. Fungal sexual spores are of the following types:

A. ascospores.
B. basidiospores.
C. sporangiospores.
D. conidia.
E. zygospores.

A. . . . . .   B. . . . . .   C. . . . . .   D. . . . . .   E. . . . . .

50. *Neisseria gonorrhoeae*:

A. is a Gram-positive diplococcus.
B. will grow on New York City medium.
C. gives a positive oxidase test.
D. ferments glucose and maltose.
E. can be resistant to penicillin by producing β-lactamase.

A. . . . . .   B. . . . . .   C. . . . . .   D. . . . . .   E. . . . . .

51. The following statements concern *Streptococcus pyogenes*:

A. *Streptococcus pyogenes* is the Lancefield group C streptococcus.
B. M protein is a major virulence factor.
C. *Streptococcus pyogenes* is sensitive to bacitracin.
D. streptolysin O causes haemolysis of blood agar.
E. *Streptococcus pyogenes* is α-haemolytic.

A. . . . . .   B. . . . . .   C. . . . . .   D. . . . . .   E. . . . . .

52. The following discoveries are paired with their discoverers:

    A.   Gram stain – Pasteur.
    B.   acid-fast stain – James Fast.
    C.   *Mycobacterium leprae* – Hansen.
    D.   salvarsan – Ehrlich.
    E.   streptomycin – Waksman.

       A. . . . . .   B. . . . . .   C. . . . . .   D. . . . . .   E. . . . . .

53. The following characteristics are found in prokaryotes and eukaryotes:

    A.   nuclear membrane – prokaryote.
    B.   more than one chromosome – eukaryote.
    C.   sterol-containing cytoplasmic membrane – eukaryote.
    D.   nucleolus – prokaryote.
    E.   ribosomes – prokaryote.

       A. . . . . .   B. . . . . .   C. . . . . .   D. . . . . .   E. . . . . .

54. Bacterial siderophores are important in bacterial pathogenesis because:

    A.   they inhibit phagocytosis.
    B.   they help extract iron from host tissues.
    C.   they enable the bacterium to adhere to host tissue.
    D.   they are regulated by the iron content in the bacterium's immediate environment.
    E.   they are high-molecular weight enzymes.

       A. . . . . .   B. . . . . .   C. . . . . .   D. . . . . .   E. . . . . .

55. The following are defences to infection found at mucosal surfaces:

    A.   secretory IgA.
    B.   microflora.
    C.   exotoxin.
    D.   mucus.
    E.   lysozyme.

       A. . . . . .   B. . . . . .   C. . . . . .   D. . . . . .   E. . . . . .

56. The following statements concern epidemiology:

   A. the mosquito is a mechanical vector in the transmission of malaria.
   B. an infectious agent acquired from the mother's vaginal flora is an example of vertical transmission.
   C. the term 'endemic' means the occurrence of cases clearly in excess of expectancy.
   D. a healthy carrier is a person with an infection that has been inapparent throughout its course.
   E. fomites are involved in direct transmission.

   A. . . . . .   B. . . . . .   C. . . . . .   D. . . . . .   E. . . . . .

57. Enzymes associated with *Neisseria gonorrhoeae* are:

   A. oxidase.
   B. lecithinase.
   C. IgA protease.
   D. streptokinase.
   E. hyaluronidase.

   A. . . . . .   B. . . . . .   C. . . . . .   D. . . . . .   E. . . . . .

58. The following statements concern *Bacillus* species:

   A. *Bacillus cereus* produces two enterotoxins.
   B. *Bacillus cereus* colonies have a 'medusa head' appearance.
   C. oedema factor is a component of the exotoxin of *Bacillus anthracis*.
   D. anthrax is primarily a disease of rats.
   E. spores of the anthrax bacillus are produced only in animal host tissues.

   A. . . . . .   B. . . . . .   C. . . . . .   D. . . . . .   E. . . . . .

✓ **59.** The following parasites are recognized causes of diarrhoea:

   A. *Entamoeba coli.*
   B. *Cryptosporidium parvum.*
   C. *Toxoplasma gondii.*
   D. *Giardia lamblia.*
   E. *Entamoeba histolytica.*

   A. . . . . .   B. . . . . .   C. . . . . .   D. . . . . .   E. . . . . .

60. The following statements concern HIV infection:

    A.   the T4 cell count starts to decline immediately after infection.

    B.   most HIV infections are transmitted by sexual contact.

    C.   the principal serological test is an ELISA test to detect HIV antigen in serum.

    D.   HIV is a retrovirus.

    E.   zidovudine is the primary drug used in treatment.

    A. . . . .   B. . . . .   C. . . . .   D. . . . .   E. . . . .

61. *Listeria monocytogenes*:

    A.   is a Gram-negative rod.

    B.   is β-haemolytic on blood agar.

    C.   is a recognized cause of meningitis.

    D.   is a recognized cause of endocarditis.

    E.   is associated with soft cheeses.

    A. . . . .   B. . . . .   C. . . . .   D. . . . .   E. . . . .

62. The following statements concern *Vibrio cholerae*:

    A.   *Vibrio cholerae* is a curved, non-motile rod.

    B.   *Vibrio cholerae* can be cultured on TCBS agar.

    C.   *Vibrio cholerae* non-01 strains do not cause gastroenteritis.

    D.   cholera enterotoxin affects adenyl cyclase.

    E.   the major cause of death in cholera is a toxin-mediated heart failure.

    A. . . . .   B. . . . .   C. . . . .   D. . . . .   E. . . . .

63. The following statements concern mycoplasmas and L-forms:

    A.   L-forms can revert back to the parental form by producing a cell wall.

    B.   mycoplasma cell membranes contain sterols.

    C.   mycoplasmas are characteristically sensitive to penicillin.

    D.   *Ureaplasma urealyticum* fails to hydrolyse urea.

    E.   L-forms can be obtained from nearly all bacterial species.

    A. . . . .   B. . . . .   C. . . . .   D. . . . .   E. . . . .

✓ **64.** *Chlamydia* species are recognized causes of:

    A. lymphogranuloma venereum.
    B. trachoma.
    C. farmers' lung.
    D. Q fever.
    E. pelvic inflammatory disease.

    A. . . . . .   B. . . . . .   C. . . . . .   D. . . . . .   E. . . . . .

✓ **65.** *Staphylococcus epidermidis* infections have a recognized association with the following:

    A. neonatal meningitis.
    B. prosthetic hips.
    C. Tenckhoff catheters.
    D. CSF shunts.
    E. prosthetic heart valves.

    A. . . . . .   B. . . . . .   C. . . . . .   D. . . . . .   E. . . . . .

66. *Acanthamoeba* species are recognized causes of:

    A. granulomatous encephalitis.
    B. dysentery.
    C. keratitis.
    D. vaginitis.
    E. liver abscess.

    A. . . . . .   B. . . . . .   C. . . . . .   D. . . . . .   E. . . . . .

67. The following antibiotics are effective prophylaxis in contacts of a case of meningococcal meningitis:

    A. penicillin.
    B. erythromycin.
    C. ciprofloxacin.
    D. ceftriaxone.
    E. rifampicin.

    A. . . . . .   B. . . . . .   C. . . . . .   D. . . . . .   E. . . . . .

68. The following statements concern bacteriuria of pregnancy:

  A. most women with bacteriuria of pregnancy are asymptomatic.
  B. clinical symptoms of pyelonephritis occur in 5% of untreated bacteriuric women.
  C. there is an association between bacteriuria of pregnancy and premature births.
  D. ciprofloxacin can be used to treat bacteriuria of pregnancy.
  E. treatment reduces the risk of pyelonephritis.

  A. . . . . .   B. . . . . .   C. . . . . .   D. . . . . .   E. . . . . .

69. Monitoring of blood levels of the following antimicrobial agents is routinely required:

  A. benzylpenicillin.
  B. gentamicin.
  C. amphotericin B.
  D. vancomycin.
  E. erythromycin.

  A. . . . . .   B. . . . . .   C. . . . . .   D. . . . . .   E. . . . . .

70. *Bacteroides fragilis* is a major pathogen in the following infections:

  A. endocarditis.
  B. peritonitis.
  C. brain abscess.
  D. liver abscess.
  E. meningitis.

  A. . . . . .   B. . . . . .   C. . . . . .   D. . . . . .   E. . . . . .

71. The following antibiotics inhibit protein synthesis in ribosomes in the bacterial cell:

  A. ciprofloxacin.
  B. polymixin.
  C. gentamicin.
  D. erythromycin.
  E. tetracycline.

  A. . . . . .   B. . . . . .   C. . . . . .   D. . . . . .   E. . . . . .

72. *Campylobacter jejuni:*

    A.   is an s-shaped spirally curved rod.
    B.   is microaerophilic.
    C.   causes gastroenteritis.
    D.   is usually sensitive to erythromycin.
    E.   will not grow in culture at 43°C.

      A. . . . .   B. . . . . .   C. . . . .   D. . . . .   E. . . . . .

73. The following statements concern actinomycosis:

    A.   cervicofacial actinomycosis is the most common form of actinomycosis.
    B.   pus contains 'sulphur granules'.
    C.   *Actinomyces israelii* is a facultative anaerobe.
    D.   *Actinomyces* species are branching fungi.
    E.   penicillin can be used to treat actinomycosis.

      A. . . . .   B. . . . . .   C. . . . .   D. . . . .   E. . . . . .

74. The following statements concern amoebic dysentery:

    A.   the transparent tape-slide method is useful in diagnosis.
    B.   the usual pathogen is *Entamoeba coli.*
    C.   motile cysts may be seen in fresh stools.
    D.   amoebic abscesses most often occur in the lung.
    E.   metronidazole can be used to treat amoebic dysentery.

      A. . . . .   B. . . . . .   C. . . . .   D. . . . .   E. . . . . .

75. The following antibiotics can be used to treat typhoid fever:

    A.   ciprofloxacin.
    B.   gentamicin.
    C.   amoxycillin.
    D.   chloramphenicol.
    E.   cefuroxime.

      A. . . . .   B. . . . . .   C. . . . .   D. . . . .   E. . . . . .

Histopathology – Questions

✓ **76.** Cell death:

    A. by apoptosis is energy dependent.

    B. as a result of viral infection implies integration of viral DNA into host DNA.

    C. in ischaemia is associated with decreased intracellular free calcium.

    D. induced by cytotoxic T lymphocytes occurs through the action of soluble mediators.

    E. is associated with loss of selective permeability.

    A. . . . .   B. . . . . .   C. . . . . .   D. . . . . .   E. . . . . .

✓ **77.** Necrosis:

    A. of fibrinoid type is found at the base of healing skin wounds.

    B. following thrombosis of a renal artery is of colliquative (liquefactive) type.

    C. can be recognized histologically by nuclear changes.

    D. normally elicits an inflammatory response.

    E. may be followed by the deposition of calcium.

    A. . . . .   B. . . . . .   C. . . . . .   D. . . . . .   E. . . . . .

✓ **78.** The following are examples of X-linked genetic disorders:

    A. haemochromatosis.

    B. red/green colour blindness.

    C. adrenogenital syndrome.

    D. Duchenne muscular dystrophy.

    E. myotonic dystrophy.

    A. . . . .   B. . . . . .   C. . . . . .   D. . . . . .   E. . . . . .

79. The following are examples of hyperplasia:

A. thickening of the left ventricle in aortic stenosis.
B. gynaecomastia.
C. replacement of respiratory columnar epithelium by squamous epithelium in response to smoking.
D. diabetic retinopathy.
E. polycythemia due to chronic hypoxia.

A. . . . . .   B. . . . . .   C. . . . . .   D. . . . . .   E. . . . . .

80. The following endothelial cell products are antithrombotic agents:

A. platelet-activating factor.
B. plasminogen activator inhibitors.
C. prostacyclin.
D. thrombomodulin.
E. endothelin-1.

A. . . . . .   B. . . . . .   C. . . . . .   D. . . . . .   E. . . . . .

81. The following are associated with disseminated intravascular coagulation:

A. septicaemia.
B. von Willebrand's disease.
C. carcinoma of the pancreas.
D. amniotic fluid embolism.
E. burns.

A. . . . . .   B. . . . . .   C. . . . . .   D. . . . . .   E. . . . . .

82. In endotoxic shock:

A. there is peripheral vasoconstriction.
B. there is frequently a normal cardiac output.
C. haemodynamic changes are mediated in part by tumour necrosis factor α.
D. there is often metabolic alkalosis.
E. there is a mortality rate of over 50%.

A. . . . . .   B. . . . . .   C. . . . . .   D. . . . . .   E. . . . . .

83. The following compounds mediate increased vascular permeability in acute inflammation:

- A. C5a.
- B. interleukin-6.
- C. histamine.
- D. leukotrienes C_4, D_4 and E_4.
- E. interleukin-8.

A. . . . . .   B. . . . . .   C. . . . . .   D. . . . . .   E. . . . . .

84. Complement activation:

- A. can occur via the classic pathway by the action of snake venoms.
- B. occurs via the alternative pathway through the action of endotoxins.
- C. leads to the generation of the membrane attack complex C5b6789.
- D. via the classic pathway is controlled by C1 inhibitor.
- E. can occur through the action of bradykinin.

A. . . . . .   B. . . . . .   C. . . . . .   D. . . . . .   E. . . . . .

85. The following are causes of granulomatous inflammation:

- A. *Staphylococcus aureus* infections.
- B. beryllium.
- C. *Mycobacterium avium intracellulare.*
- D. measles virus infection.
- E. sarcoidosis.

A. . . . . .   B. . . . . .   C. . . . . .   D. . . . . .   E. . . . . .

86. Vitamin A:

- A. deficiency occurs in chronic renal failure.
- B. deficiency is associated with impairment of blood clotting.
- C. deficiency is associated with squamous metaplasia of the conjunctiva (xerophthalmia).
- D. toxicity may be associated with liver cirrhosis.
- E. is carcinogenic in high doses.

A. . . . . .   B. . . . . .   C. . . . . .   D. . . . . .   E. . . . . .

87. During the formation of granulation tissue:

    A. the first matrix protein to be laid down is collagen type I.
    B. proliferating blood vessels lie parallel to the wound surface.
    C. production of collagens by fibroblasts is mediated by transforming growth factor β.
    D. myofibroblasts serve to contract the wound.
    E. epithelioid macrophages are the predominant cell type.

    A. . . . . .   B. . . . . .   C. . . . . .   D. . . . . .   E. . . . . .

88. The following factors are known to impair healing of skin wounds:

    A. vitamin D deficiency.
    B. diabetes mellitus.
    C. poor blood supply.
    D. Cushing's syndrome.
    E. hypomagnesaemia.

    A. . . . . .   B. . . . . .   C. . . . . .   D. . . . . .   E. . . . . .

89. The following are examples of type II hypersensitivity reactions:

    A. autoimmune thrombocytopaenic purpura.
    B. extrinsic asthma.
    C. rhesus incompatibility.
    D. Goodpasture's syndrome.
    E. Mantoux reaction.

    A. . . . . .   B. . . . . .   C. . . . . .   D. . . . . .   E. . . . . .

90. The following are examples of organ-specific autoimmune diseases:

    A. Addison's disease.
    B. Conn's syndrome.
    C. rheumatoid arthritis.
    D. myaesthenia gravis.
    E. type I diabetes mellitus.

    A. . . . . .   B. . . . . .   C. . . . . .   D. . . . . .   E. . . . . .

91. Amyloid:

A. is an extracellular accumulation of protein arranged as cross-striated fibrils.
B. in primary amyloidosis is of AA type.
C. associated with multiple myeloma is of AL type.
D. may occur as a complication of haemodialysis treatment.
E. is a cause of cardiomyopathy.

A. . . . . .   B. . . . . .   C. . . . . .   D. . . . . .   E. . . . . .

92. Iron overload:

A. is a feature of Wilson's disease.
B. may be associated with cardiac failure.
C. is a complication of a thalassaemia.
D. may be complicated by Cushing's syndrome.
E. associated with genetic haemochromatosis is seen more frequently in females than in males.

A. . . . . .   B. . . . . .   C. . . . . .   D. . . . . .   E. . . . . .

93. In the cell cycle.

A. DNA synthesis occurs throughout G_1 and S phases.
B. cells move from G_0 into G_1 under the action of peptide growth factors.
C. M (mitosis) is the phase with the longest duration.
D. transition from G_2 to M requires the action of phosphokinases.
E. G_0 phase represents a non-proliferating state.

A. . . . . .   B. . . . . .   C. . . . . .   D. . . . . .   E. . . . . .

94. The following are examples of benign tumours:

A. seminoma.
B. leiomyoma.
C. squamous papilloma.
D. glioblastoma multiforme.
E. neurofibroma.

A. . . . . .   B. . . . . .   C. . . . . .   D. . . . . .   E. . . . . .

95. Detection of the following molecules in serum can be used as tumour markers:

  A. carcinoembryonic antigen.
  B. thyroglobulin.
  C. tumour necrosis factor α.
  D. C reactive protein.
  E. βHCG.

  A. . . . . . B. . . . . . C. . . . . . D. . . . . . E. . . . . .

96. Viruses have been implicated in the pathogenesis of the following human tumours:

  A. nasopharyngeal carcinoma.
  B. Hodgkin's disease.
  C. colonic carcinoma.
  D. hepatocellular carcinoma.
  E. cervical carcinoma.

  A. . . . . . B. . . . . . C. . . . . . D. . . . . . E. . . . . .

97. The following are thought to contribute to tumour invasion:

  A. increased expression of cadherins.
  B. altered expression of integrins.
  C. decreased expression of matrix metalloproteinases.
  D. increased expression of growth factor receptors.
  E. induction of angiogenesis.

  A. . . . . . B. . . . . . C. . . . . . D. . . . . . E. . . . . .

98. The following environmental agents have been implicated in the development of malignant liver tumours:

  A. asbestos.
  B. benzo(a)pyrene.
  C. vinyl chloride.
  D. aflatoxins.
  E. nitrosamines.

  A. . . . . . B. . . . . . C. . . . . . D. . . . . . E. . . . . .

99. The following are examples of tumour suppressor genes:

    A. c-*myc*.
    B. H-*ras*.
    C. p53.
    D. retinoblastoma gene (RB-1).
    E. *bcl2*.

    A. . . . . B. . . . . C. . . . . D. . . . . E. . . . .

100. The following are non-metastatic effects of some malignant tumours:

    A. Cushing's syndrome.
    B. hypercalcaemia.
    C. iron deficiency anaemia.
    D. dermatomyositis.
    E. acanthosis nigricans.

    A. . . . . B. . . . . C. . . . . D. . . . . E. . . . .

101. Dystrophic calcification is found in the following conditions:

    A. primary hyperparathyroidism.
    B. atheroma.
    C. carcinomatosis with bony metastases.
    D. sarcoidosis.
    E. fat necrosis.

    A. . . . . B. . . . . C. . . . . D. . . . . E. . . . .

102. The following are risk factors for the development of atheroma:

    A. diabetes mellitus.
    B. elevated high density lipoprotein levels.
    C. type B behaviour pattern.
    D. systemic hypertension.
    E. anaemia.

    A. . . . . B. . . . . C. . . . . D. . . . . E. . . . .

103. The following are causes of secondary hypertension:

    A. chronic glomerulonephritis.
    B. phaeochromocytoma.
    C. primary biliary cirrhosis.
    D. Klinefelter's syndrome.
    E. Conn's syndrome.

    A. . . . .   B. . . . .   C. . . . .   D. . . . .   E. . . . .

104. The following are examples of vasculitis:

    A. Wegener's granulomatosis.
    B. Henoch–Schönlein purpura.
    C. senile purpura.
    D. dermatitis herpetiformis.
    E. Buerger's disease.

    A. . . . .   B. . . . .   C. . . . .   D. . . . .   E. . . . .

105. Aortic aneurysms:

    A. in syphilis are most commonly seen in the arch of the aorta.
    B. in the abdominal aorta are most frequently seen above the level of the renal arteries.
    C. of the thoracic aorta can be complicated by recurrent laryngeal nerve palsy.
    D. can be complicated by high output cardiac failure.
    E. occur more commonly in females than in males.

    A. . . . .   B. . . . .   C. . . . .   D. . . . .   E. . . . .

106. The following are causes of left ventricular hypertrophy:

    A. recurrent pulmonary thromboembolism.
    B. renal artery stenosis.
    C. tricuspid valve disease.
    D. coarctation of the aorta.
    E. aortic valve incompetence.

    A. . . . .   B. . . . .   C. . . . .   D. . . . .   E. . . . .

107. Myocardial infarction:

 A. is a complication of polyarteritis nodosa.
 B. is associated with elevated serum alkaline phosphatase.
 C. is associated with Dressler's syndrome.
 D. is most commonly caused by occlusion of the left circumflex coronary artery.
 E. can lead to mitral valve incompetence.

 A. . . . . .   B. . . . . .   C. . . . . .   D. . . . . .   E. . . . . .

108. The following are causes of myocarditis:

 A. Takayasu's disease.
 B. giant cell arteritis.
 C. Coxsackie A virus.
 D. toxoplasmosis.
 E. rheumatic fever.

 A. . . . . .   B. . . . . .   C. . . . . .   D. . . . . .   E. . . . . .

109. Rheumatic fever:

 A. occurs as a sequel to staphylococcal infections.
 B. is associated with Aschoff bodies in the heart.
 C. is associated with erythema marginatum.
 D. leads to chronic heart failure in over 50% of cases.
 E. is mediated by type II hypersensitivity reaction.

 A. . . . . .   B. . . . . .   C. . . . . .   D. . . . . .   E. . . . . .

110. The following are cyanotic forms of congenital heart disease:

 A. Fallot's tetralogy.
 B. patent ductus arteriosus.
 C. coarctation of the aorta.
 D. truncus arteriosus.
 E. transposition of the great vessels.

 A. . . . . .   B. . . . . .   C. . . . . .   D. . . . . .   E. . . . . .

111. The following are causes of pericarditis:

    A. hepatic failure.
    B. rheumatoid arthritis.
    C. tuberculosis.
    D. carcinoma of bronchus.
    E. hyperthyroidism.

    A. . . . . .   B. . . . . .   C. . . . . .   D. . . . . .   E. . . . . . .

112. Emphysema:

    A. is abnormal and irreversible dilatation of the bronchi.
    B. in α_1- antitrypsin deficiency is of centrilobular type.
    C. is a feature of coal workers' pneumoconiosis.
    D. of interstitial type is most frequently seen in trauma.
    E. of centrilobular type can lead to right ventricular failure.

    A. . . . . .   B. . . . . .   C. . . . . .   D. . . . . .   E. . . . . . .

113. Pneumonia:

    A. caused by *Klebsiella* infection is most commonly seen in infancy.
    B. of lobar type can be seen in legionnaires' disease.
    C. caused by cytomegalovirus is a complication of bone marrow transplantation.
    D. in measles infection is characterized by the presence of giant cells in the lung.
    E. of lobar type in pneumococcal infection is complicated by pulmonary fibrosis in 30% of cases.

    A. . . . . .   B. . . . . .   C. . . . . .   D. . . . . .   E. . . . . . .

114. The following are causes of diffuse pulmonary fibrosis:

    A. busulphan treatment.
    B. exposure to asbestos.
    C. cigarette smoking.
    D. lymphangitis carcinomatosis.
    E. bird fancier's lung.

    A. . . . . .   B. . . . . .   C. . . . . .   D. . . . . .   E. . . . . . .

115. Carcinoma of the bronchus:

    A.   may be complicated by hyponatraemia.
    B.   is most frequently of small cell (oat cell) type.
    C.   is a complication of asbestos exposure.
    D.   may be associated with Cushing's syndrome.
    E.   arising at the periphery of the lung is most commonly of squamous cell type.

    A. . . . . .   B. . . . . .   C. . . . . .   D. . . . . .   E. . . . . .

116. Carcinoma of the oesophagus:

    A.   arising in the upper third of the oesophagus is most commonly adenocarcinoma.
    B.   is rare in the Far East.
    C.   is associated with cigarette smoking.
    D.   is a complication of achalasia.
    E.   usually causes death by widespread metastases.

    A. . . . . .   B. . . . . .   C. . . . . .   D. . . . . .   E. . . . . .

117. Chronic gastritis:

    A.   type B is caused by mycobacterial infections.
    B.   type A is associated with pernicious anaemia.
    C.   of lymphocytic type is associated with *Helicobacter* infection.
    D.   associated with bile reflux is characterized by foveolar hyperplasia and oedema.
    E.   is commonly caused by fungal infection.

    A. . . . . .   B. . . . . .   C. . . . . .   D. . . . . .   E. . . . . .

118. Coeliac disease:

    A.   commonly leads to malabsorption.
    B.   is associated with increase in villous length.
    C.   is associated with crypt hyperplasia.
    D.   is associated with pollen hypersensitivity.
    E.   may be complicated by small intestinal lymphoma.

    A. . . . . .   B. . . . . .   C. . . . . .   D. . . . . .   E. . . . . .

119. Pseudomembranous colitis:

    A. is associated with *Helicobacter* infection.
    B. is characterized by granulomatous tissue reaction.
    C. is associated with the use of lincomycin.
    D. can be diagnosed by the detection of toxins in faecal samples.
    E. is a premalignant condition.

    A. . . . .   B. . . . . .   C. . . . . .   D. . . . . .   E. . . . . .

120. Ulcerative colitis:

    A. can affect any part of the gastrointestinal tract.
    B. is associated with primary sclerosing cholangitis.
    C. is more common in the ascending colon than in the rectum.
    D. is a common cause of malabsorption.
    E. is associated with ankylosing spondylitis.

    A. . . . .   B. . . . .   C. . . . .   D. . . . .   E. . . . . .

121. The following are causes of malabsorption:

    A. chronic pancreatitis.
    B. staphylococcal food poisoning.
    C. abetalipoproteinaemia.
    D. diverticular disease.
    E. giardiasis.

    A. . . . .   B. . . . . .   C. . . . . .   D. . . . . .   E. . . . . .

122. Carcinoma of the colon:

    A. is a complication of familial adenomatous polyposis.
    B. is most frequently of squamous type.
    C. can be graded according to Dukes' classification.
    D. is a complication of ulcerative colitis.
    E. is more common in Third World than in industrialized countries.

    A. . . . .   B. . . . . .   C. . . . . .   D. . . . . .   E. . . . . .

123. The following are harmful effects of excess alcohol:

    A. steatohepatitis.
    B. cholecystitis.
    C. acute pancreatitis.
    D. subacute combined degeneration of the spinal cord.
    E. cardiomyopathy.

    A. . . . . .　B. . . . . .　C. . . . . .　D. . . . . .　E. . . . . .

124. The following are causes of cirrhosis of the liver:

    A. hepatitis A infection.
    B. acute paracetamol intoxication.
    C. hepatitis C infection.
    D. leptospirosis.
    E. α_1-antitrypsin deficiency.

    A. . . . . .　B. . . . . .　C. . . . . .　D. . . . . .　E. . . . . .

125. Primary biliary cirrhosis:

    A. is more frequently seen in males than in females.
    B. is associated with Sjögren's syndrome.
    C. is characterized by the presence of circulating antinuclear antibodies.
    D. is characterized by granulomatous destruction of bile ducts.
    E. commonly leads to hypercholesterolaemia.

    A. . . . . .　B. . . . . .　C. . . . . .　D. . . . . .　E. . . . . .

126. Fatty liver (steatosis) is a feature of the following conditions:

    A. Reye's syndrome.
    B. autoimmune chronic hepatitis.
    C. alcoholic liver disease.
    D. type 2 diabetes mellitus.
    E. protein energy malnutrition.

    A. . . . . .　B. . . . . .　C. . . . . .　D. . . . . .　E. . . . . .

127. Type 1 diabetes mellitus:

    A. occurs most frequently in elderly patients.
    B. is associated with circulating anti-islet cell antibodies.
    C. is associated with obesity.
    D. is associated with loss of α cells in the pancreatic islets.
    E. is associated with an increased risk of ischaemic heart disease.

    A. . . . . .   B. . . . . .   C. . . . . .   D. . . . . .   E. . . . . .

128. The following are causes of acute pancreatitis:

    A. hypothermia.
    B. alcohol abuse.
    C. cystic fibrosis.
    D. gallstones.
    E. trauma.

    A. . . . . .   B. . . . . .   C. . . . . .   D. . . . . .   E. . . . . .

129. The following are causes of granulomatous lymphadenopathy:

    A. toxoplasmosis.
    B. Epstein Barr virus infection.
    C. Crohn's disease.
    D. rheumatoid arthritis.
    E. sarcoidosis.

    A. . . . . .   B. . . . . .   C. . . . . .   D. . . . . .   E. . . . . .

130. In Hodgkin's disease:

    A. the most common histological subtype is lymphocyte-depleted Hodgkin's disease.
    B. disease involving nodes on both sides of the diaphragm in the absence of extranodal tumour is stage 3.
    C. the lymphocyte predominant subtype carries a good prognosis.
    D. Reed–Sternberg cells are regarded to be the malignant element.
    E. the lymphocytic component is monoclonal.

    A. . . . . .   B. . . . . .   C. . . . . .   D. . . . . .   E. . . . . .

131. T cell lymphomas are associated with:

    A.   mycosis fungoides.
    B.   human papilloma virus.
    C.   HTLV-1 retrovirus.
    D.   coeliac disease.
    E.   amyloidosis of AL type.

    A. . . . . .   B. . . . . .   C. . . . . .   D. . . . . .   E. . . . . .

132. Raised intracranial pressure:

    A.   leads to systemic hypotension.
    B.   is associated with tachycardia.
    C.   leads to papilloedema.
    D.   may cause brain stem haemorrhage.
    E.   may lead to pulmonary oedema.

    A. . . . . .   B. . . . . .   C. . . . . .   D. . . . . .   E. . . . . .

133. The following are causes of primary hydrocephalus:

    A.   cerebral infarction in the territory supplied by the middle cerebral artery.
    B.   Arnold Chiari malformation.
    C.   colloid cyst of third ventricle.
    D.   Parkinson's disease.
    E.   aqueduct stenosis.

    A. . . . . .   B. . . . . .   C. . . . . .   D. . . . . .   E. . . . . .

134. The following are examples of demyelinating disorders:

    A.   Alzheimer's disease.
    B.   progressive multifocal leucoencephalopathy.
    C.   multiple sclerosis.
    D.   Huntington's disease.
    E.   hepatic encephalopathy.

    A. . . . . .   B. . . . . .   C. . . . . .   D. . . . . .   E. . . . . .

135. Acute diffuse proliferative glomerulonephritis:

    A. is associated with malaria.
    B. is associated with specific subtypes of β-haemolytic streptococci.
    C. is characterized histologically by diffuse thickening of the glomerular basement membranes.
    D. is characterized by the presence of circulating antibasement membrane antibody.
    E. in children progresses to crescentic glomerulonephritis in over 50%.

    A. . . . . .   B. . . . . .   C. . . . . .   D. . . . . .   E. . . . . .

136. The following conditions predispose to the development of acute pyelonephritis:

    A. infective endocarditis.
    B. vesicoureteric reflux.
    C. gout.
    D. diabetes mellitus.
    E. amyloidosis.

    A. . . . . .   B. . . . . .   C. . . . . .   D. . . . . .   E. . . . . .

137. Carcinoma of the bladder:

    A. is usually of adenocarcinoma type.
    B. is associated with schistosomiasis.
    C. may be complicated by hydroureter.
    D. is found with increased frequency in coal workers.
    E. are frequently papillary.

    A. . . . . .   B. . . . . .   C. . . . . .   D. . . . . .   E. . . . . .

138. Teratoma of testis:

    A. occurs most frequently after the age of 50 years.
    B. is usually benign.
    C. may be associated with raised serum α- fetoprotein.
    D. is usually radiosensitive.
    E. is of germ cell origin.

    A. . . . . .   B. . . . . .   C. . . . . .   D. . . . . .   E. . . . . .

139. Paget's disease of bone:

    A. is usually associated with normal serum calcium levels.
    B. is caused by vitamin D deficiency.
    C. may be complicated by cardiac failure.
    D. predisposes to the development of malignant bone tumours.
    E. is characterized by decreased osteoclast activity.

    A. . . . . .   B. . . . . .   C. . . . . .   D. . . . . .   E. . . . . .

140. Ewing's sarcoma:

    A. is seen most frequently in children and adolescents.
    B. is a tumour of chondrocytes.
    C. is associated with raised urinary catecholamines.
    D. frequently shows a reciprocal translocation in cytogenetic analyses.
    E. is treated by local resection alone.

    A. . . . . .   B. . . . . .   C. . . . . .   D. . . . . .   E. . . . . .

141. Rheumatoid arthritis:

    A. is more frequent in males than in females.
    B. is associated with hyperplasia of the synovium.
    C. is associated with circulating immune complexes.
    D. shows a strong association with HLA- B27.
    E. is a component of Felty's syndrome.

    A. . . . . .   B. . . . . .   C. . . . . .   D. . . . . .   E. . . . . .

142. Cervical intraepithelial neoplasia:

    A. is associated with human papilloma virus infection.
    B. is a precursor lesion for invasive adenocarcinoma.
    C. can be detected by cytology.
    D. is rare in virgins.
    E. is associated with *in utero* exposure to diethylstilboestrol.

    A. . . . . .   B. . . . . .   C. . . . . .   D. . . . . .   E. . . . . .

143. Carcinoma of the breast:

    A.   may present with Paget's disease of the nipple.
    B.   most frequently occurs in the lower inner quadrant of the breast.
    C.   is responsive to hormone treatment in over 30% of patients.
    D.   is most frequently of infiltrating lobular type.
    E.   of ductal carcinoma *in situ* type has a ten-year survival rate of over 90%.

    A. . . . . .   B. . . . . .   C. . . . . .   D. . . . . .   E. . . . . .

144. Hashimoto's thyroiditis:

    A.   is associated with exophthalmos.
    B.   carries an increased risk of the development of lymphoma.
    C.   is associated with circulating antimicrosomal antibodies in over 80% of patients.
    D.   is characterized histologically by the presence of Hürthle cells and a lymphocytic infiltrate.
    E.   is a result of dietary iodine deficiency.

    A. . . . . .   B. . . . . .   C. . . . . .   D. . . . . .   E. . . . . .

145. Papillary carcinoma of thyroid:

    A.   occurs most frequently in the elderly.
    B.   is a cause of hyperthyroidism.
    C.   is derived from the C cells of the thyroid.
    D.   frequently spreads to cervical lymph nodes.
    E.   often shows dystrophic calcification.

    A. . . . . .   B. . . . . .   C. . . . . .   D. . . . . .   E. . . . . .

146. Primary hyperparathyroidism:

    A.   is a complication of chronic renal failure.
    B.   may occur as part of multiple endocrine neoplasia syndromes.
    C.   leads to the formation of renal calculi.
    D.   is most frequently caused by parathyroid carcinoma.
    E.   is associated with osteitis fibrosa cystica.

    A. . . . . .   B. . . . . .   C. . . . . .   D. . . . . .   E. . . . . .

✓ **147.** The following are examples of bullous skin disorders:

    A.   erythema nodosum.
    B.   dermatitis herpetiformis.
    C.   pemphigus vulgaris.
    D.   lichen planus.
    E.   psoriasis.

     A. . . . .   B. . . . . .   C. . . . . .   D. . . . . .   E. . . . . .

148. The following are premalignant squamous lesions in the skin:

    A.   squamous papilloma.
    B.   seborrhoeic keratosis.
    C.   actinic keratosis.
    D.   keratoacanthoma.
    E.   Bowen's disease.

     A. . . . .   B. . . . . .   C. . . . . .   D. . . . . .   E. . . . . .

149. The following are examples of viral skin disorders:

    A.   molluscum contagiosum.
    B.   impetigo.
    C.   herpes gestationis.
    D.   verruca vulgaris.
    E.   condyloma accuminatum.

     A. . . . .   B. . . . . .   C. . . . . .   D. . . . . .   E. . . . . .

✓ **150.** The following methods can be used to detect specific proteins in tissues:

    A.   immunohistochemistry.
    B.   Northern blotting.
    C.   polymerase chain reaction.
    D.   Western blotting.
    E.   *in situ* hybridization.

     A. . . . .   B. . . . . .   C. . . . . .   D. . . . . .   E. . . . . .

Clinical Biochemistry – Questions

151. The following are causes of selective water depletion:

    A. coma.
    B. treatment with lithium salts.
    C. vasopressin administration.
    D. diabetic ketoacidosis.
    E. dysphagia.

    A. . . . . .   B. . . . . .   C. . . . . .   D. . . . . .   E. . . . . .

152. The following statements concern sodium:

    A. sodium is the principal extracellular cation.
    B. aldosterone stimulates sodium secretion into the distal convoluted tubule.
    C. urinary sodium excretion decreases in postoperative patients.
    D. hyponatraemia always indicates sodium depletion.
    E. sodium retention occurs in Cushing's syndrome.

    A. . . . . .   B. . . . . .   C. . . . . .   D. . . . . .   E. . . . . .

153. The following statements concern serum osmolality:

    A. serum osmolality is a measure of the concentration of solute per litre of serum.
    B. sodium and its associated anions determine approximately 50% of the serum osmolality.
    C. increased serum osmolality inhibits ADH secretion.
    D. serum osmolality is normal if hyponatraemia is caused by hyperproteinaemia.
    E. serum osmolality is raised in psychogenic polydipsia.

    A. . . . . .   B. . . . . .   C. . . . . .   D. . . . . .   E. . . . . .

154. The following are features of an Addisonian crisis:

    A.   low serum ACTH concentrations.
    B.   hypernatraemia.
    C.   hyperkalaemia.
    D.   metabolic alkalosis.
    E.   uraemia.

    A. . . . .   B. . . . . .   C. . . . . .   D. . . . . .   E. . . . . .

155. The following statements concern potassium:

    A.   insulin infusion increases potassium uptake into muscle and liver cells.
    B.   decreased plasma potassium concentrations cause decreased aldosterone secretion.
    C.   hyperkalaemia causes tall, peaked T waves on an ECG.
    D.   metabolic acidosis is a recognized complication of potassium deficiency.
    E.   hypokalaemia is a complication of treatment with the diuretic amiloride.

    A. . . . .   B. . . . . .   C. . . . . .   D. . . . . .   E. . . . . .

156. Aldosterone secretion is stimulated by:

    A.   angiotensinogen I.
    B.   ACTH.
    C.   hypernatraemia.
    D.   recumbency.
    E.   hypovolaemia.

    A. . . . .   B. . . . . .   C. . . . . .   D. . . . . .   E. . . . . .

157. The following test results are typical of non-respiratory (metabolic) acidosis:

    A.   blood pH 7.32.
    B.   plasma bicarbonate 12 mmol/l.
    C.   blood $P\text{co}_2$ 7.4 kPa.
    D.   plasma potassium 3.1 mmol/l.
    E.   blood $P\text{o}_2$ 8.0 kPa.

    A. . . . .   B. . . . . .   C. . . . . .   D. . . . . .   E. . . . . .

158. Lactic acidosis:

A. causes metabolic acidosis with a normal anion gap.
B. is a recognized complication of treating type II diabetes mellitus with sulphonylurea drugs.
C. occurs in medium chain acyl-CoA dehydrogenase (MCAD) deficiency.
D. is a recognized complication of hepatic failure.
E. occurs in McArdle's syndrome (type V glycogen storage disease).

A. . . . . .   B. . . . . .   C. . . . . .   D. . . . . .   E. . . . . .

159. Type I renal tubular acidosis:

A. is always an inherited disorder.
B. causes hyperkalaemia.
C. is caused by a tubular defect in bicarbonate reabsorption.
D. causes increased serum chloride.
E. causes osteomalacia.

A. . . . . .   B. . . . . .   C. . . . . .   D. . . . . .   E. . . . . .

160. The following substances are used to measure glomerular filtration rate:

A. creatinine.
B. urea.
C. inulin.
D. EDTA.
E. para-aminohippuric acid.

A. . . . . .   B. . . . . .   C. . . . . .   D. . . . . .   E. . . . . .

161. The following statements concern urea:

A. it is synthesized in the kidney.
B. plasma concentrations are independent of dietary protein intake.
C. plasma concentrations may be raised after a gastrointestinal bleed.
D. uraemia is a recognized complication of congestive cardiac failure.
E. normal plasma values exclude impaired renal function.

A. . . . . .   B. . . . . .   C. . . . . .   D. . . . . .   E. . . . . .

162. The following are properties of the kidney:

    A. gluconeogenesis.
    B. erythropoietin production.
    C. excretion of unconjugated bilirubin.
    D. synthesis of 25-hydroxycholecalciferol.
    E. secretion of angiotensinogen.

       A...... B...... C...... D...... E......

163. The following occur in chronic renal failure:

    A. positive H^+ balance.
    B. toxaemia which is the result of urea retention.
    C. oliguria.
    D. infertility.
    E. increased serum alkaline phosphatase activity.

       A...... B...... C...... D...... E......

164. The following are recognized features of the nephrotic syndrome:

    A. hypoalbuminaemia.
    B. increased total serum thyroxine levels.
    C. hypercholesterolaemia.
    D. decreased serum α_2-globulin levels.
    E. proteinuria.

       A...... B...... C...... D...... E......

165. The following statements concern renal tract calculi:

    A. most patients with a single calcium-containing stone do not form another.
    B. calcium phosphate precipitation is favoured by acid urine.
    C. oxalate stones may complicate intestinal disease.
    D. uric acid stones are radio-opaque.
    E. cystinuria is a single amino acid excretion abnormality.

       A...... B...... C...... D...... E......

166. The following statements concern calcium:

    A. approximately 50% of serum calcium is in the form of free ions (Ca^{2+}).

    B. the main calcium-binding protein in serum is albumin.

    C. Ca^{2+} levels are decreased by acidosis.

    D. Ca^{2+} levels control neuromuscular excitability.

    E. Ca^{2+} is an intracellular second messenger of hormone action.

    A. . . . . .   B. . . . . .   C. . . . . .   D. . . . . .   E. . . . . .

167. Parathyroid hormone (PTH):

    A. secretion is regulated by serum ionized calcium (Ca^{2+}) concentration.

    B. acts on hormone receptors on the cell membranes of target organs.

    C. decreases renal tubular reabsorption of calcium.

    D. decreases renal tubular reabsorption of bicarbonate.

    E. decreases renal tubular reabsorption of phosphate.

    A. . . . . .   B. . . . . .   C. . . . . .   D. . . . . .   E. . . . . .

168. The following are causes of hypocalcaemia:

    A. end-stage renal disease.

    B. osteoporosis.

    C. hypoparathyroidism.

    D. magnesium deficiency.

    E. acute pancreatitis.

    A. . . . . .   B. . . . . .   C. . . . . .   D. . . . . .   E. . . . . .

169. The following are causes of hypercalcaemia:

    A. secondary hyperparathyroidism.

    B. carcinoma of the bronchus.

    C. sarcoidosis.

    D. osteomalacia.

    E. thiazide diuretics.

    A. . . . . .   B. . . . . .   C. . . . . .   D. . . . . .   E. . . . . .

170. Hypophosphataemia occurs in:

    A.   vitamin D intoxication.
    B.   patients being given parenteral nutrition.
    C.   patients recovering from diabetic ketoacidosis.
    D.   Paget's disease of the bone.
    E.   acromegaly.

    A. . . . .   B. . . . . .   C. . . . . .   D. . . . . .   E. . . . . .

171. The following are causes of hypomagnesaemia:

    A.   myocardial infarction.
    B.   parathyroidectomy.
    C.   alcoholism.
    D.   chronic renal failure.
    E.   diabetic ketoacidosis.

    A. . . . .   B. . . . . .   C. . . . . .   D. . . . . .   E. . . . . .

172. The following statements concern lipoproteins:

    A.   very low density lipoproteins arise from chylomicrons.
    B.   low density lipoproteins contain apolipoprotein AI.
    C.   cholesterol is the major lipid of low density lipoprotein.
    D.   chylomicrons are cleared from the circulation by lipoprotein lipase.
    E.   high density lipoprotein is a source of apolipoproteins for chylomicrons and very low density lipoprotein.

    A. . . . .   B. . . . . .   C. . . . . .   D. . . . . .   E. . . . . .

173. The following statements concern hyperlipidaemia:

    A.   familial hypercholesterolaemia is an autosomal recessive condition.
    B.   eruptive xanthomas are a clinical feature of familial hypercholesterolaemia.
    C.   type III hyperlipoproteinaemia (familial dysbetalipoproteinaemia) is associated with the apolipoprotein E2/E2 phenotype.
    D.   raised circulating low density lipoprotein cholesterol levels are a risk factor for coronary heart disease.
    E.   lipoprotein lipase deficiency causes type I hyperlipidaemia (chylomicronaemia syndrome).

    A. . . . .   B. . . . . .   C. . . . . .   D. . . . . .   E. . . . . .

174. The following are causes of secondary hyperlipidaemia:

    A. treatment with β-blocking drugs.
    B. alcohol abuse.
    C. diabetes insipidus.
    D. hyperthyroidism.
    E. cholestasis.

    A. . . . .   B. . . . . .   C. . . . . .   D. . . . . .   E. . . . . .

175. The following statements concern obesity:

    A. in obese patients the resting metabolic rate is decreased.
    B. basal serum insulin levels are raised in obesity.
    C. obesity is an independent risk factor for coronary heart disease.
    D. the incidence of hypertension is increased in obesity.
    E. the prevalence of rheumatoid arthritis is increased in obesity.

    A. . . . .   B. . . . . .   C. . . . . .   D. . . . . .   E. . . . . .

176. Insulin:

    A. exerts its action through a specific receptor in cell nuclei.
    B. inhibits the release of non-esterified fatty acids (NEFA) from
        adipose tissue.
    C. increases ketone body production.
    D. increases amino acid release from muscle.
    E. inhibits glycogenolysis.

    A. . . . .   B. . . . . .   C. . . . . .   D. . . . . .   E. . . . . .

177. In type 1 diabetes mellitus:

    A. there is an absence of A (α) cells in the islets of Langerhans.
    B. is associated with specific HLA antigens.
    C. is rarely associated with circulating islet cell antibodies at
        presentation.
    D. rarely presents in childhood.
    E. ketosis is often present at diagnosis.

    A. . . . .   B. . . . . .   C. . . . . .   D. . . . . .   E. . . . . .

178. Type 2 (non-insulin-dependent) diabetes mellitus:

  A. never occurs in patients less than 40 years of age.
  B. is associated with weight loss.
  C. in identical twins has an almost 100% concordance rate.
  D. insulin secretion is normal or slightly reduced.
  E. never requires treatment with insulin.

  A. . . . . .   B. . . . . .   C. . . . . .   D. . . . . .   E. . . . . .

179. The following occur in diabetic ketoacidosis:

  A. leucocytosis.
  B. hypernatraemia.
  C. decreased secretion of counterregulatory hormones.
  D. Kussmaul breathing.
  E. hypovolaemia.

  A. . . . . .   B. . . . . .   C. . . . . .   D. . . . . .   E. . . . . .

180. Hyperosmolar non-ketotic coma (HONK):

  A. may be the presenting feature of type 2 diabetes.
  B. is rarely fatal.
  C. is commonly accompanied by hypernatraemia.
  D. is never associated with increased blood ketone levels.
  E. does not require treatment with insulin.

  A. . . . . .   B. . . . . .   C. . . . . .   D. . . . . .   E. . . . . .

181. The following are causes of hypoglycaemia:

  A. thiazide therapy.
  B. retroperitoneal sarcoma.
  C. Addison's disease.
  D. reaction to alcohol.
  E. nicotinic acid therapy.

  A. . . . . .   B. . . . . .   C. . . . . .   D. . . . . .   E. . . . . .

182. C-Peptide:

    A.   is secreted in equimolar amounts with insulin.
    B.   the amino acid sequences are identical between species.
    C.   is low in serum in type I diabetes.
    D.   serum levels are elevated by sulphonylureas.
    E.   serum levels are increased in insulinoma.

    A. . . . .   B. . . . . .   C. . . . . .   D. . . . . .   E. . . . . .

183. The following statements concern type I glycogen storage disease:

    A.   it is due to deficiency of amylo-(1,6)-glucosidase (debrancher enzyme).
    B.   the liver is the only tissue affected.
    C.   is a cause of hypoglycaemia.
    D.   causes hepatomegaly.
    E.   causes ketoacidosis.

    A. . . . .   B. . . . . .   C. . . . . .   D. . . . . .   E. . . . . .

184. The following statements concern galactosaemia:

    A.   galactosaemia is caused by a single enzyme defect.
    B.   cataracts are a clinical feature.
    C.   aminoaciduria occurs in galactosaemia.
    D.   reducing substances occur in urine.
    E.   jaundice is a recognized complication.

    A. . . . .   B. . . . . .   C. . . . . .   D. . . . . .   E. . . . . .

185. The following statements concern carbohydrate digestion and absorption:

    A.   in the UK the majority of carbohydrate intake is in the form of glucose.
    B.   pancreatic amylase hydrolyses $\alpha(1\rightarrow6)$ linkages between glucose units in starch.
    C.   lactose is hydrolysed to glucose and fructose.
    D.   fructose is actively transported across the jejunal mucosa.
    E.   sugars which are not digested in the small intestine are fermented in the colon to products which include hydrogen.

    A. . . . .   B. . . . . .   C. . . . . .   D. . . . . .   E. . . . . .

186. The following statements concern amino acids and proteins:

    A.   dietary protein absorption occurs entirely in the form of amino acids.

    B.   malabsorption of cystine, ornithine, arginine and lysine occurs in cystinuria.

    C.   phenylalanine is an essential amino acid.

    D.   the proteolytic enzyme trypsin acts best at an acid pH.

    E.   increased urinary nitrogen excretion occurs after a surgical operation.

    A. . . . . .   B. . . . . .   C. . . . . .   D. . . . . .   E. . . . . .

187. The following statements concern vitamins:

    A.   vitamin E is an antioxidant.

    B.   follicular keratosis occurs in vitamin A deficiency.

    C.   riboflavin is a coenzyme for decarboxylation and transamination reactions.

    D.   flavin adenine dinucleotide contains nicotinic acid.

    E.   folic acid is necessary for nucleic acid synthesis.

    A. . . . . .   B. . . . . .   C. . . . . .   D. . . . . .   E. . . . . .

188. The following are complications of parenteral nutrition:

    A.   hyperglycaemia.

    B.   fatty liver.

    C.   lipaemia.

    D.   hyponatraemia.

    E.   metabolic acidosis.

    A. . . . . .   B. . . . . .   C. . . . . .   D. . . . . .   E. . . . . .

189. Classic phenylketonuria:

    A.   is caused by phenylalanine hydroxylase deficiency.

    B.   may be detected by enzyme assay in cultured fibroblasts.

    C.   is a sex-linked condition.

    D.   is characterized by high blood tyrosine levels.

    E.   is treated by dietary therapy the objective of which is to maintain blood phenylalanine levels below normal.

    A. . . . . .   B. . . . . .   C. . . . . .   D. . . . . .   E. . . . . .

190. The following test procedures may be used to detect malabsorption due to pancreatic disease:

    A. ammonium chloride loading.
    B. triglyceride tolerance.
    C. xylose absorption.
    D. hydrogen breath analysis.
    E. ^{14}C-PABA excretion test.

    A. ..... B. ..... C. ..... D. ..... E. .....

191. Hypolactasia:

    A. is rare in non-Caucasian adults.
    B. causes reduced faecal pH in children.
    C. occurs transiently in gastroenteritis.
    D. occurs in coeliac disease.
    E. always causes increased breath hydrogen excretion following an oral lactose load.

    A. ..... B. ..... C. ..... D. ..... E. .....

192. Pancreatitis:

    A. serum amylase activities >5 times the upper limit of normal are diagnostic.
    B. leads to reduced urinary amylase excretion.
    C. is never complicated by diabetes mellitus.
    D. may cause methaemalbuminaemia.
    E. may be precipitated by severe hypercholesterolaemia.

    A. ..... B. ..... C. ..... D. ..... E. .....

193. The following statements concern paraproteins:

    A. paraproteins are immunoglobulins produced by T cells.
    B. all molecules in a paraprotein are identical.
    C. a paraprotein is excluded if a band is not seen on serum electrophoresis.
    D. paraproteins may be benign.
    E. all paraproteins are detected in the γ region on electrophoresis.

    A. ..... B. ..... C. ..... D. ..... E. .....

194. α₁-Antitrypsin:

    A.   is an acute phase reactant.
    B.   is a protease inhibitor.
    C.   deficiency is most commonly the result of homozygosity for the
        M allele.
    D.   deficiency is associated with emphysema.
    E.   deficiency is associated with cirrhosis in childhood.

    A. . . . .   B. . . . .   C. . . . .   D. . . . .   E. . . . .

195. The following statements concern serum albumin:

    A.   albumin concentration is high in portal cirrhosis.
    B.   albumin transports unconjugated bilirubin in blood.
    C.   albumin is raised in prolonged venous stasis.
    D.   oedema is a constant feature of analbuminaemia.
    E.   hypoalbuminaemic states are associated with secondary
        hyperaldosteronism.

    A. . . . .   B. . . . .   C. . . . .   D. . . . .   E. . . . .

196. The following are functions of the liver:

    A.   synthesis of immunoglobulins.
    B.   synthesis of both primary and secondary bile acids.
    C.   gluconeogenesis.
    D.   ketone body production.
    E.   synthesis of urobilinogen.

    A. . . . .   B. . . . .   C. . . . .   D. . . . .   E. . . . .

197. Serum bilirubin:

    A.   is predominantly conjugated in normal subjects.
    B.   is decreased by phenobarbitone administration.
    C.   is unconjugated in Gilbert's disease.
    D.   is conjugated in haemolytic jaundice.
    E.   is conjugated in the Dubin–Johnson syndrome.

    A. . . . .   B. . . . .   C. . . . .   D. . . . .   E. . . . .

198. The following serum enzymes are useful indicators of liver cell damage:

    A.   creatine kinase.
    B.   aspartate aminotransferase.
    C.   alanine aminotransferase.
    D.   hydroxybutyrate dehydrogenase.
    E.   alkaline phosphatase.

    A. . . . . .   B. . . . . .   C. . . . . .   D. . . . . .   E. . . . . .

199. The following are features of cholestasis:

    A.   increased serum conjugated bilirubin.
    B.   increased urinary urobilinogen.
    C.   increased serum γ-glutamyl transpeptidase.
    D.   osteomalacia.
    E.   increased blood ammonia levels.

    A. . . . . .   B. . . . . .   C. . . . . .   D. . . . . .   E. . . . . .

200. The following are recognized features of Wilson's disease:

    A.   increased hepatic copper content.
    B.   aminoaciduria.
    C.   decreased serum caeruloplasmin concentrations.
    D.   increased serum copper concentrations.
    E.   diabetes mellitus.

    A. . . . . .   B. . . . . .   C. . . . . .   D. . . . . .   E. . . . . .

201. Serum cholinesterase:

    A.   is reduced in chronic liver disease.
    B.   is reduced by anaesthesia.
    C.   deficiency causes scoline apnoea.
    D.   is reduced in renal disease.
    E.   is reduced in organophosphate poisoning.

    A. . . . . .   B. . . . . .   C. . . . . .   D. . . . . .   E. . . . . .

202. Serum tartrate-labile acid phosphatase:

    A.   increases in benign prostatic hypertrophy.

    B.   is increased by prostatic palpation in normal subjects.

    C.   is generally elevated in patients with disseminated prostatic carcinoma.

    D.   may be high in breast carcinoma.

    E.   may be high in Gaucher's disease.

A. . . . . .   B. . . . . .   C. . . . . .   D. . . . . .   E. . . . . .

203. The following statements concern cardiac enzymes and myocardial infarction:

    A.   increased serum creatine kinase (CK) activity in a patient with characteristic chest pain is diagnostic of myocardial infarction.

    B.   the cardiac isoenzyme of CK (CK-MB) increases later than total CK following myocardial infarction.

    C.   the time of maximum increase in CK following myocardial infarction is approximately 12 hours.

    D.   continuing increased serum CK activity suggests infarct extension.

    E.   AST activity remains elevated for 5 to 6 days.

A. . . . . .   B. . . . . .   C. . . . . .   D. . . . . .   E. . . . . .

204. Growth hormone secretion:

    A.   occurs in short bursts.

    B.   is inhibited by stress.

    C.   is stimulated by glucose.

    D.   is stimulated by interleukin-1.

    E.   is controlled by two regulatory hypothalamic hormones.

A. . . . . .   B. . . . . .   C. . . . . .   D. . . . . .   E. . . . . .

205. The following statements concern acromegaly:

    A.   a clinical feature is overgrowth of skin and subcutaneous tissue.

    B.   it is the result of a basophil tumour.

    C.   it may cause diabetes insipidus.

    D.   it may be accompanied by glucose intolerance.

    E.   it may be accompanied by galactorrhoea.

A. . . . . .   B. . . . . .   C. . . . . .   D. . . . . .   E. . . . . .

206. The following statements concern gonadal function:

A. in women, there is a large peak in serum FSH just prior to ovulation.
B. in men, interstitial cell-stimulating hormone promotes development of seminiferous tubules.
C. serum gonadotrophin levels are low in primary gonadal failure.
D. clomiphene administration increases secretion of gonadotrophin-releasing hormone.
E. levels of LH and FSH fall after the menopause.

A. . . . . .   B. . . . . .   C. . . . . .   D. . . . . .   E. . . . . .

207. The following statements concern antidiuretic hormone (ADH):

A. serum ADH levels increase in shock, despite reduced serum osmolality.
B. inappropriate ADH secretion is a recognized feature of carcinoma of the bronchus.
C. chlorpropamide potentiates ADH action.
D. general anaesthesia inhibits ADH secretion.
E. ADH increases active water transport in the collecting duct of the kidney.

A. . . . . .   B. . . . . .   C. . . . . .   D. . . . . .   E. . . . . .

208. The following are causes of hyperprolactinaemia:

A. venepuncture.
B. chlorpromazine administration.
C. progestogens.
D. craniopharyngioma.
E. hyperthyroidism.

A. . . . . .   B. . . . . .   C. . . . . .   D. . . . . .   E. . . . . .

209. The following statements concern the thyroid gland:

A. thyroid hormones are required for normal growth.
B. the intracellular effects of thyroid hormones are mediated by binding with cell membrane receptors.
C. hyperthyroidism is associated with increased sex hormone binding globulin levels.
D. hypothyroidism can be excluded if the serum TSH is normal.
E. hyperthyroidism in Graves' disease is caused by excessive pituitary production of TSH.

A. . . . . .   B. . . . . .   C. . . . . .   D. . . . . .   E. . . . . .

210. The following statements concern serum free thyroxine concentrations:

A. increased during pregnancy.
B. decreased by androgens.
C. increased by amiodarone.
D. always raised in thyrotoxicosis.
E. is unaffected by severe non-thyroidal illness.

A. . . . . .   B. . . . . .   C. . . . . .   D. . . . . .   E. . . . . .

211. The following are actions of glucocorticoids:

A. enhancement of gluconeogenesis.
B. inhibition of diuresis.
C. increase of blood lymphocyte counts.
D. anti-inflammatory effects.
E. hypotensive effect.

A. . . . . .   B. . . . . .   C. . . . . .   D. . . . . .   E. . . . . .

212. The following statements concern Cushing's syndrome:

A. 20% of cases are the result of pituitary-dependent adrenocortical hyperplasia.
B. Cushing's syndrome may cause amenorrhoea.
C. excess cortisol secretion caused by an adrenal adenoma is suppressed by high dose dexamethasone.
D. Cushing's syndrome may be differentiated from simple obesity by the response to insulin-induced hypoglycaemia.
E. hypokalaemia is a feature of Cushing's syndrome caused by ectopic production of ACTH.

A. . . . . .   B. . . . . .   C. . . . . .   D. . . . . .   E. . . . . .

213. Congenital adrenal hyperplasia:

   A. is most often caused by 11β-hydroxylase deficiency.
   B. salt loss is a rare feature.
   C. may cause hypertension.
   D. may cause hypokalaemia.
   E. may present as infertility.

   A. . . . . . B. . . . . . C. . . . . . D. . . . . . E. . . . . .

214. The following are causes of secondary amenorrhoea:

   A. abnormalities of sex chromosomes.
   B. hyperprolactinaemia.
   C. Kallman's syndrome.
   D. anorexia nervosa.
   E. Sheehan's syndrome.

   A. . . . . . B. . . . . . C. . . . . . D. . . . . . E. . . . . .

215. The following biochemical changes occur in pregnancy:

   A. increased serum alkaline phosphatase.
   B. decreased plasma urea.
   C. decreased serum cholesterol.
   D. decreased serum cortisol.
   E. increased incidence of impaired glucose tolerance.

   A. . . . . . B. . . . . . C. . . . . . D. . . . . . E. . . . . .

216. The following endocrine conditions are causes of hypertension:

   A. phaeochromocytoma.
   B. primary hyperparathyroidism.
   C. hypothyroidism.
   D. Conn's syndrome.
   E. non-insulin-dependent diabetes mellitus (NIDDM).

   A. . . . . . B. . . . . . C. . . . . . D. . . . . . E. . . . . .

217.   Ethanol:

  A.   induces hepatic synthesis of γ-glutamyl transpeptidase.
  B.   reduces serum HDL-cholesterol concentrations.
  C.   induces hyperglycaemia.
  D.   induces hypercortisolism.
  E.   inhibits gastric acid secretion.

  A. . . . . .   B. . . . . .   C. . . . . .   D. . . . . .   E. . . . . .

218.   The following are features of lead poisoning:

  A.   increased urinary excretion of δ-aminolaevulinic acid.
  B.   peripheral neuropathy.
  C.   leucocytosis.
  D.   polycythaemia.
  E.   aminoaciduria.

  A. . . . . .   B. . . . . .   C. . . . . .   D. . . . . .   E. . . . . .

219.   The following are features of salicylate intoxication:

  A.   tinnitus.
  B.   metabolic acidosis.
  C.   liver failure.
  D.   impaired renal function.
  E.   treatment is with a specific antidote.

  A. . . . . .   B. . . . . .   C. . . . . .   D. . . . . .   E. . . . . .

220.   In paracetamol poisoning:

  A.   liver damage is caused by hepatic necrosis.
  B.   the toxic metabolites are glucuronide and sulphate conjugates of the drug.
  C.   hypoglycaemia may occur.
  D.   renal failure is a recognized complication.
  E.   blood levels are best determined within 4 hours of an overdose.

  A. . . . . .   B. . . . . .   C. . . . . .   D. . . . . .   E. . . . . .

221. The following are features of the carcinoid syndrome:

    A.   increased urinary excretion of homovanillic acid.
    B.   increased urinary excretion of 5-hydroxyindole acetic acid.
    C.   decreased platelet serotonin levels.
    D.   paroxysmal hypotension.
    E.   diarrhoea.

    A. .....   B. .....   C. .....   D. .....   E. .....

222. The following cause hyperuricaemia:

    A.   pre-eclampsia.
    B.   Lesch–Nyhan syndrome.
    C.   myeloproliferative disorders.
    D.   treatment with colchicine.
    E.   Fanconi syndrome.

    A. .....   B. .....   C. .....   D. .....   E. .....

223. The following are features of acute intermittent porphyria:

    A.   increased faecal excretion of protoporphyrin.
    B.   increased urinary excretion of porphobilinogen.
    C.   cutaneous photosensitivity.
    D.   neuropathies.
    E.   sensitivity to oestrogens.

    A. .....   B. .....   C. .....   D. .....   E. .....

224. The following statements concern biochemical tests:

    A.   if values have a Gaussian distribution the range of the mean ± 2 standard deviations includes 66% of the population.
    B.   the sensitivity of a test measures the incidence of patients free of disease.
    C.   the specificity of a test measures the incidence of patients positive for a disease.
    D.   the efficiency of a test measures the number of correct results.
    E.   the accuracy of a test measures its reproducibility.

    A. .....   B. .....   C. .....   D. .....   E. .....

225. The following statements concern reference ranges:

    A.   they include all values expected in a healthy population.

    B.   they always have a Gaussian distribution.

    C.   they are independent of analytical methods.

    D.   they may differ between sexes and with age.

    E.   they indicate the variation in results which may occur in a single individual.

    A. . . . .   B. . . . . .   C. . . . . .   D. . . . . .   E. . . . . .

Haematology – Questions

226. Microcytic anaemia often occurs in:

    A. iron deficiency.
    B. thalassaemia.
    C. sickle cell trait.
    D. renal failure.
    E. anaemia of chronic disorder.

       A. . . . .   B. . . . . .   C. . . . . .   D. . . . . .   E. . . . . .

227. In the normal newborn:

    A. the MCV is lower than in adults.
    B. adult haemoglobin is undetectable.
    C. the Kleihauer test is usually negative.
    D. the haemoglobin concentration is higher than in adults.
    E. circulating nucleated red cells may be found.

       A. . . . .   B. . . . . .   C. . . . . .   D. . . . . .   E. . . . . .

228. Haemolytic disease of the newborn:

    A. is inevitable if the mother is Rh D negative.
    B. can be prevented by exchange transfusion of the infant.
    C. can be treated by phototherapy.
    D. can be caused by hereditary spherocytosis.
    E. is more likely to be caused by G6PD deficiency in the Far East.

       A. . . . .   B. . . . . .   C. . . . . .   D. . . . . .   E. . . . . .

229. Haemolytic disease of the newborn has decreased in incidence because:

    A.   postpartum use of anti-D, when indicated, is widespread.
    B.   family sizes are smaller.
    C.   blood transfusion in the population is less common.
    D.   younger women are less likely to be sensitized.
    E.   premature babies now have an improved survival rate.

       A. . . . .   B. . . . . .   C. . . . . .   D. . . . . .   E. . . . . .

230. Folic acid deficiency:

    A.   can cause megaloblastic anaemia.
    B.   is often associated with severe neuropathy.
    C.   can cause coeliac disease.
    D.   is always associated with a raised MCV.
    E.   can occur in vegetarians.

       A. . . . .   B. . . . . .   C. . . . . .   D. . . . . .   E. . . . . .

231. Pernicious anaemia:

    A.   is best treated by daily injections of vitamin B_{12}.
    B.   is caused by lack of intrinsic factor.
    C.   can be caused by surgical removal of the terminal ileum.
    D.   will respond to erythropoietin.
    E.   is diagnosed by the Schilling test.

       A. . . . .   B. . . . . .   C. . . . . .   D. . . . . .   E. . . . . .

232. Severe bacterial infections:

    A.   can cause neutrophil leucocytosis.
    B.   can cause leukopenia.
    C.   may cause myelocytes to appear in the blood.
    D.   often cause lymphocytosis.
    E.   can mimic leukaemia.

       A. . . . .   B. . . . . .   C. . . . . .   D. . . . . .   E. . . . . .

233. Idiopathic thrombocytopenic purpura:

    A.   is usually a fatal disorder if untreated.
    B.   is caused by bone marrow failure.
    C.   may respond to treatment with steroids.
    D.   is best treated with splenectomy.
    E.   may recover spontaneously.

    A. . . . .   B. . . . . .   C. . . . . .   D. . . . . .   E. . . . . .

234. Thrombocytosis of $>1000 \times 10^9/l$:

    A.   may follow infections or surgery.
    B.   always needs specific treatment.
    C.   can cause cerebrovascular accidents.
    D.   may be associated with a bleeding tendency.
    E.   excludes a diagnosis of polycythaemia rubra vera.

    A. . . . .   B. . . . . .   C. . . . . .   D. . . . . .   E. . . . . .

235. Haemophilia A:

    A.   usually presents with purpura in the first year of life.
    B.   is inherited in an autosomal recessive pattern.
    C.   is associated with a prolonged bleeding time.
    D.   is best treated with cryoprecipitate.
    E.   is caused by low factor IX levels.

    A. . . . .   B. . . . . .   C. . . . . .   D. . . . . .   E. . . . . .

236. Disseminated intravascular coagulation is a recognized complication of:

    A.   retained placenta.
    B.   septicaemia.
    C.   contraceptive pill overdose.
    D.   von Willebrand's disease.
    E.   acute promyelocytic leukaemia.

    A. . . . .   B. . . . . .   C. . . . . .   D. . . . . .   E. . . . . .

237.   Anticoagulation with warfarin in a patient with deep vein thrombosis is:

   A.   monitored by the INR.
   B.   fine-tuned by daily adjustments of the dose.
   C.   fine-tuned by administering vitamin K.
   D.   carried out to prevent stroke.
   E.   carried out to prevent pulmonary embolus.

   A. . . . . .   B. . . . . .   C. . . . . .   D. . . . . .   E. . . . . .

238.   Autoimmune haemolytic anaemia:

   A.   may be caused by eating fava beans.
   B.   causes conjugated hyperbilirubinaemia.
   C.   is associated with non-Hodgkin's lymphoma.
   D.   may respond to cholecystectomy.
   E.   may respond to steroid therapy.

   A. . . . . .   B. . . . . .   C. . . . . .   D. . . . . .   E. . . . . .

239.   Coombs negative haemolytic anaemia may be:

   A.   associated with spherocytes in the blood.
   B.   caused by artificial heart valves.
   C.   inherited.
   D.   caused by sulphonamides.
   E.   immune mediated.

   A. . . . . .   B. . . . . .   C. . . . . .   D. . . . . .   E. . . . . .

240.   Howell–Jolly bodies are:

   A.   sometimes known as Heinz bodies.
   B.   small granules of iron within red cells.
   C.   denatured haemoglobin inclusions.
   D.   found after splenectomy.
   E.   a sign of parasitic infection of red cells.

   A. . . . . .   B. . . . . .   C. . . . . .   D. . . . . .   E. . . . . .

241. The direct Coombs test:

   A. detects antibody on red cell surfaces.
   B. is the usual way to perform ABO blood grouping.
   C. is used to gauge the severity of haemolysis.
   D. is never positive in Rh haemolytic disease of the newborn.
   E. is usually positive after blood transfusion.

   A. . . . . . B. . . . . . C. . . . . . D. . . . . . E. . . . . .

242. T lymphocytes:

   A. are so called because they are processed by the thyroid.
   B. have a very short life span.
   C. secrete antibodies.
   D. are the major defence mechanism against bacteria.
   E. are undetectable in the newborn.

   A. . . . . . B. . . . . . C. . . . . . D. . . . . . E. . . . . .

243. B lymphocytes:

   A. are phagocytes.
   B. reject foreign tissue grafts.
   C. express immunoglobulins on their surface.
   D. may be infected by Epstein–Barr virus.
   E. respond to phytohaemagglutinin (PHA).

   A. . . . . . B. . . . . . C. . . . . . D. . . . . . E. . . . . .

244. Hypogammaglobulinaemia is well recognized in:

   A. chronic lymphocytic leukaemia.
   B. multiple myeloma.
   C. non-Hodgkin's lymphoma.
   D. chronic granulocytic leukaemia.
   E. chronic granulomatous disease.

   A. . . . . . B. . . . . . C. . . . . . D. . . . . . E. . . . . .

245.   Infusion of high dose IgG is of value in:

   A.   ITP.
   B.   common variable immunodeficiency.
   C.   acute renal failure.
   D.   autoimmune haemolytic anaemia (AIHA).
   E.   asthma.

   A. . . . . .   B. . . . . .   C. . . . . .   D. . . . . .   E. . . . . .

246.   Chronic granulocytic leukaemia is characterized by:

   A.   large numbers of monocytes.
   B.   proliferation of neutrophils.
   C.   inheritance of the Philadelphia chromosome.
   D.   proliferation of platelets.
   E.   an extra chromosome 21.

   A. . . . . .   B. . . . . .   C. . . . . .   D. . . . . .   E. . . . . .

247.   Oncogenes:

   A.   are found in normal cells.
   B.   may be activated in cancer cells.
   C.   are part of the cytosol.
   D.   are viruses.
   E.   are specialized mitochondria.

   A. . . . . .   B. . . . . .   C. . . . . .   D. . . . . .   E. . . . . .

248.   The *bcr/abl* hybrid gene:

   A.   is characteristic of chronic granulocytic leukaemia.
   B.   is characteristic of polycythaemia rubra vera.
   C.   may be found in acute leukaemia.
   D.   is located on chromosome 22.
   E.   is an acquired abnormality.

   A. . . . . .   B. . . . . .   C. . . . . .   D. . . . . .   E. . . . . .

249. The cells of chronic lymphoid leukaemias may be:

    A. T lymphocytes.
    B. B lymphocytes.
    C. plasma cells.
    D. NK lymphocytes.
    E. lymphoblasts.

    A. . . . . .   B. . . . . . .   C. . . . . D. . . . . . .   E. . . . . .

250. The following are well described in chronic lymphatic leukaemia:

    A. splenomegaly.
    B. increased tendency to bacterial infections.
    C. priapism.
    D. lymphadenopathy.
    E. meningeal infiltration with leukaemia.

    A. . . . . .   B. . . . . . .   C. . . . . .   D. . . . . . .   E. . . . . .

251. Polycythaemia rubra vera is associated with:

    A. increased erythropoietin levels.
    B. increased red cell mass.
    C. decreased Po_2 of arterial blood.
    D. renal tumours.
    E. increased bone marrow cellularity.

    A. . . . . .   B. . . . . . .   C. . . . . .   D. . . . . . .   E. . . . . .

252. Normal adult haemoglobin contains:

    A. alpha chains.
    B. beta chains.
    C. gamma chains.
    D. kappa chains.
    E. lambda chains.

    A. . . . . .   B. . . . . . .   C. . . . . .   D. . . . . . .   E. . . . . .

253. Acute lymphoblastic leukaemia is:

    A.   more common in children than in adults.
    B.   the most common cause of bone marrow failure in children.
    C.   caused by cytomegalovirus.
    D.   treated with chlorambucil.
    E.   usually a proliferation of B-precursor lymphoid cells.

    A. . . . . .   B. . . . . .   C. . . . . .   D. . . . . .   E. . . . . .

254. In acute myeloblastic leukaemia the blasts usually:

    A.   are positive with Sudan black.
    B.   have obvious nucleoli.
    C.   have more cytoplasm than lymphoblasts.
    D.   have normal karyotypes.
    E.   can ingest bacteria.

    A. . . . . .   B. . . . . .   C. . . . . .   D. . . . . .   E. . . . . .

255. Bone marrow transplantation is important in first-line treatment of:

    A.   acute myeloblastic leukaemia.
    B.   childhood acute lymphoblastic leukaemia.
    C.   aplastic anaemia.
    D.   chronic ITP.
    E.   chronic granulocytic leukaemia.

    A. . . . . .   B. . . . . .   C. . . . . .   D. . . . . .   E. . . . . .

256. AIDS is associated with:

    A.   elevated CD4 positive lymphocytes.
    B.   decreased CD8 positive lymphocytes.
    C.   pneumatosis cystoides intestinalis.
    D.   intravenous drug abuse.
    E.   lymphoma.

    A. . . . . .   B. . . . . .   C. . . . . .   D. . . . . .   E. . . . . .

257. The following are important in the management of AIDS:

    A. acyclovir,
    B. AZT.
    C. HVZ.
    D. cytosine arabinoside.
    E. thioguanine.

    A. . . . . . B. . . . . . C. . . . . . D. . . . . . E. . . . . .

258. Myeloma is:

    A. a malignant proliferation of myelocytes.
    B. associated with bone disease.
    C. associated with renal impairment.
    D. more often found in the elderly.
    E. associated with increased plasma viscosity.

    A. . . . . . B. . . . . . C. . . . . . D. . . . . . E. . . . . .

259. Immunoelectrophoresis of plasma proteins is usually performed to:

    A. identify hypogammaglobulinaemia.
    B. exclude immunodeficiency.
    C. identify the nature of an M band.
    D. detect hypoalbuminaemia.
    E. detect antiviral antibodies.

    A. . . . . . B. . . . . . C. . . . . . D. . . . . . E. . . . . .

260. Bence-Jones protein is:

    A. albumin leaking through damaged glomeruli.
    B. free haemoglobin in the urine.
    C. heavy chain of immunoglobulin.
    D. immunoglobulin light chains.
    E. found in Fanconi's syndrome.

    A. . . . . . B. . . . . . C. . . . . . D. . . . . . E. . . . . .

261.   Treatment with heparin:

    A.   reduces blood viscosity.
    B.   causes clot lysis.
    C.   improves capillary blood flow.
    D.   is counteracted by vitamin K.
    E.   is monitored by measuring the fibrinogen level.

    A. . . . . .   B. . . . . .   C. . . . . .   D. . . . . .   E. . . . . .

262.   Red cell aplasia may be associated with:

    A.   thymoma.
    B.   human parvovirus infection.
    C.   intravenous IgG infusion.
    D.   neonatal anaemia.
    E.   a raised MCV.

    A. . . . . .   B. . . . . .   C. . . . . .   D. . . . . .   E. . . . . .

263.   The following are characteristic of beta thalassaemia trait:

    A.   microcytosis.
    B.   high serum ferritin.
    C.   raised Hb A_2.
    D.   stippled red cells.
    E.   abnormal Hb electrophoresis pattern.

    A. . . . . .   B. . . . . .   C. . . . . .   D. . . . . .   E. . . . . .

264.   Alpha thalassaemia is:

    A.   caused by excess numbers of alpha chains.
    B.   unlikely to be accompanied by iron deficiency.
    C.   sometimes found in Caucasians.
    D.   usually normocytic.
    E.   more common in Asians than in Africans.

    A. . . . . .   B. . . . . .   C. . . . . .   D. . . . . .   E. . . . . .

265. In an umbilical cord blood sample:

    A.   a haemoglobin of 13 g/dl is abnormal.
    B.   IgM is usually present.
    C.   IgM has been transferred across the placenta.
    D.   IgG is rarely present.
    E.   a haemoglobin of 18 g/dl is normal.

    A. . . . .   B. . . . . .   C. . . . . .   D. . . . . .   E. . . . . .

266. Infectious mononucleosis:

    A.   is caused by Epstein–Barr virus.
    B.   is rare in children.
    C.   is characterized by increased monocytes.
    D.   may cause splenomegaly.
    E.   may be transmitted via saliva.

    A. . . . .   B. . . . . .   C. . . . . .   D. . . . . .   E. . . . . .

267. The following are usually associated with eosinophilia:

    A.   atopy.
    B.   *Toxocara canis* infection.
    C.   *Candida albicans* infection.
    D.   threadworm infestation.
    E.   polyarteritis nodosa.

    A. . . . .   B. . . . . .   C. . . . . .   D. . . . . .   E. . . . . .

268. The risk of haemorrhage due to warfarin may be potentiated by the following:

    A.   penicillin.
    B.   aspirin.
    C.   paracetamol.
    D.   barbiturates.
    E.   allopurinol.

    A. . . . .   B. . . . . .   C. . . . . .   D. . . . . .   E. . . . . .

269. The effects of warfarin may be reduced by the following:

    A. cimetidine.
    B. oral contraceptives.
    C. non-steroidal anti-inflammatory drugs.
    D. rifampicin.
    E. vitamin K.

    A. . . . .   B. . . . . .   C. . . . . .   D. . . . . .   E. . . . . .

270. The following drugs are used to induce remission in acute lymphoblastic leukaemia:

    A. vincristine.
    B. oxymethalone.
    C. prednisolone.
    D. allopurinol.
    E. melphalan.

    A. . . . .   B. . . . . .   C. . . . . .   D. . . . . .   E. . . . . .

271. The following are well known to cause severe morbidity in patients being treated for acute lymphoblastic leukaemia:

    A. herpes zoster.
    B. cytomegalovirus.
    C. rhinovirus.
    D. measles.
    E. herpes simplex.

    A. . . . .   B. . . . . .   C. . . . . .   D. . . . . .   E. . . . . .

272. CD antigen determination is used to:

    A. ascertain red cell genotype.
    B. tissue-type prospective organ donors.
    C. investigate haemopoietic cell lineage.
    D. predict haemolytic disease of the newborn.
    E. test for allergy.

    A. . . . .   B. . . . . .   C. . . . . .   D. . . . . .   E. . . . . .

273. Monoclonal antibodies:

A. may be used *in vivo* in patients.
B. may be used as diagnostic reagents.
C. are synthetic, artificial molecules.
D. are produced by living cells.
E. are only produced in laboratories.

A. . . . . . B. . . . . . C. . . . . . D. . . . . . E. . . . . .

274. Iron deficiency is:

A. excluded by a normal serum ferritin.
B. associated with koilonychia.
C. associated with pitted nails.
D. common in one-day-old infants of iron-deficient mothers.
E. known to impair the response to vitamin B_{12} in pernicious anaemia.

A. . . . . . B. . . . . . C. . . . . . D. . . . . . E. . . . . .

275. During pregnancy:

A. the MCV usually rises.
B. the haemoglobin usually falls.
C. the plasma volume decreases.
D. the red cell mass usually rises.
E. iron deficiency is rare.

A. . . . . . B. . . . . . C. . . . . . D. . . . . . E. . . . . .

276. The following drugs are known to cause aplastic anaemia:

A. penicillin.
B. chloramphenicol.
C. tricyclic antidepressants.
D. vincristine.
E. phenylbutazone.

A. . . . . . B. . . . . . C. . . . . . D. . . . . . E. . . . . .

277.   The following may cause autoimmune haemolysis:

    A.   cephalosporin antibiotics.
    B.   methyldopa.
    C.   quinine.
    D.   sulphonamides.
    E.   paracetamol.

    A. . . . .   B. . . . . .   C. . . . . .   D. . . . . .   E. . . . . .

278.   Splenectomy:

    A.   should be followed by indefinite oral penicillin.
    B.   should be preceded by immunization against pneumococcus.
    C.   is usually associated with a rise in the platelet count.
    D.   results in circulating fragmented red cells.
    E.   causes increased susceptibility to virus infections.

    A. . . . .   B. . . . . .   C. . . . . .   D. . . . . .   E. . . . . .

279.   The following are associated with Hodgkin's disease:

    A.   fever.
    B.   weight loss.
    C.   normocytic anaemia.
    D.   eosinophilia.
    E.   itching.

    A. . . . .   B. . . . . .   C. . . . . .   D. . . . . .   E. . . . . .

280.   Non-African Burkitt's lymphoma:

    A.   is a tumour of T cells.
    B.   is usually caused by Epstein–Barr virus.
    C.   commonly affects the jaw of children.
    D.   often involves the bone marrow or central nervous system.
    E.   responds to chlorambucil.

    A. . . . .   B. . . . . .   C. . . . . .   D. . . . . .   E. . . . . .

281. The following are useful in the treatment of polycythaemia rubra vera (PRV):

    A. venesection.
    B. hyperbaric oxygen.
    C. radioactive phosphorus.
    D. busulphan.
    E. methotrexate.

    A. . . . .   B. . . . .   C. . . . .   D. . . . .   E. . . . .

282. Neutropenia of <0.5 × 10⁹/l results in increased susceptibility to infection with:

    A. bacteria.
    B. respiratory syncytial virus.
    C. *Candida albicans.*
    D. *Aspergillus* spp.
    E. *Pneumocystis carinii.*

    A. . . . .   B. . . . .   C. . . . .   D. . . . .   E. . . . .

283. Blood transfusion accidents are often the result of:

    A. difficulty in determining ABO groups of recipient/donor.
    B. difficulty in determining Rh groups of recipient/donor.
    C. clerical errors.
    D. failure to detect immune antibodies in the donor blood.
    E. incorrect blood group labelling by the Blood Transfusion Service.

    A. . . . .   B. . . . .   C. . . . .   D. . . . .   E. . . . .

284. The following are features of haemolytic anaemia:

    A. raised reticulocyte count.
    B. unconjugated hyperbilirubinaemia.
    C. bilirubinuria.
    D. increased bone marrow reticulin.
    E. raised serum alkaline phosphatase.

    A. . . . .   B. . . . .   C. . . . .   D. . . . .   E. . . . .

285. Haemoglobinuria may be caused by:

    A.   urinary tract infection.
    B.   artificial heart valves.
    C.   acute glomerulonephritis.
    D.   running marathons.
    E.   hypernephroma.

    A. . . . .   B. . . . .   C. . . . .   D. . . . .   E. . . . .

286. The abnormal genes causing the following are found on autosomes:

    A.   hereditary spherocytosis.
    B.   von Willebrand's disease.
    C.   factor IX deficiency.
    D.   factor VIII deficiency.
    E.   sickle cell disease.

    A. . . . .   B. . . . .   C. . . . .   D. . . . .   E. . . . .

287. The following are characteristic features of hereditary haemorrhagic telangiectasia (HHT):

    A.   microcytosis.
    B.   epistaxis.
    C.   haemoptysis.
    D.   arteriovenous shunts.
    E.   melaena.

    A. . . . .   B. . . . .   C. . . . .   D. . . . .   E. . . . .

288. Large numbers of spider naevi should suggest:

    A.   hereditary haemorrhagic telangiectasia.
    B.   thrombocytopenia.
    C.   possible liver disease.
    D.   inhibitors of factor VIII.
    E.   vasculitis.

    A. . . . .   B. . . . .   C. . . . .   D. . . . .   E. . . . .

289. Teardrop poikilocytes are a common feature of:

A. myelofibrosis.
B. iron deficiency.
C. renal failure.
D. megaloblastic anaemia.
E. hereditary spherocytosis.

A. . . . . .   B. . . . . .   C. . . . . .   D. . . . . .   E. . . . . .

290. The following are typical of CNS involvement with acute leukaemia:

A. cranial nerve palsy.
B. headache.
C. fever.
D. papilloedema.
E. neutrophils in the CSF.

A. . . . . .   B. . . . . .   C. . . . . .   D. . . . . .   E. . . . . .

291. Cerebrospinal fluid may be less clear than water by eye because:

A. there is a high protein content.
B. the white cell count is high.
C. the glucose concentration is high.
D. red cells are present.
E. glove powder granules have entered the bottle.

A. . . . . .   B. . . . . .   C. . . . . .   D. . . . . .   E. . . . . .

292. In cerebrospinal fluid:

A. neutrophils may be present in patients with viral meningitis.
B. up to 20 lymphocytes/μl are considered normal.
C. nucleated red cells and myelocytes suggest extramedullary haemopoiesis.
D. less than 4 white cells/μl is rare.
E. xanthochromia suggests an earlier bleed into the CSF.

A. . . . . .   B. . . . . .   C. . . . . .   D. . . . . .   E. . . . . .

293. Samples of blood for a full blood count should be collected into tubes containing:

   A. heparin.
   B. EDTA.
   C. citrate.
   D. no anticoagulant.
   E. dextran.

       A. . . . . .   B. . . . . .   C. . . . . .   D. . . . . .   E. . . . . .

294. A positive test result, when ABO grouping antisera are added to red cells, is usually denoted by:

   A. rouleaux.
   B. lysis.
   C. agglutination.
   D. colour change.
   E. clotting.

       A. . . . . .   B. . . . . .   C. . . . . .   D. . . . . .   E. . . . . .

295. Elevated D-dimers are found characteristically:

   A. in autoimmune haemolysis.
   B. in disseminated intravascular coagulation.
   C. after a pulmonary embolus.
   D. in factor VIII deficiency.
   E. in patients on long-term warfarin.

       A. . . . . .   B. . . . . .   C. . . . . .   D. . . . . .   E. . . . . .

296. Pancytopenia is a recognized presenting feature of:

   A. aplastic anaemia.
   B. Fanconi's anaemia.
   C. acute leukaemia.
   D. chronic lymphocytic leukaemia.
   E. myelodysplastic syndromes.

       A. . . . . .   B. . . . . .   C. . . . . .   D. . . . . .   E. . . . . .

297. A 1.5 litre haemorrhage one hour previously in an otherwise normal adult will often have caused:

A. anaemia.
B. microcytosis.
C. shock.
D. low serum ferritin.
E. increased iron-binding capacity.

A. . . . . . B. . . . . . C. . . . . . D. . . . . . E. . . . . .

298. Haemosiderosis commonly occurs in:

A. thalassaemia major.
B. sickle cell trait.
C. peptic ulceration.
D. myelodysplastic syndromes.
E. congenital red cell asplasia.

A. . . . . . B. . . . . . C. . . . . . D. . . . . . E. . . . . .

299. Treatment with recombinant human erythropoietin is of little value in:

A. congenital red cell aplasia.
B. aplastic anaemia.
C. chronic renal failure.
D. polycythaemia rubra vera.
E. thalassaemia major.

A. . . . . . B. . . . . . C. . . . . . D. . . . . . E. . . . . .

300. Sideroblasts are:

A. present in normal marrow.
B. reduced in iron deficiency.
C. malignant cells.
D. cells containing lead granules.
E. detected by the Prussian blue staining reaction.

A. . . . . . B. . . . . . C. . . . . . D. . . . . . E. . . . . .

ANSWERS

Medical Microbiology – Answers

1. A. T
   B. F
   C. F
   D. T
   E. F

   Cell walls of Gram-positive bacteria are less complex than those of Gram-negative bacteria, consisting mainly of peptidoglycan and very little lipid. This cell wall structure makes Gram-positive bacteria more sensitive to penicillin and less resistant to lysozyme. Spore-forming bacteria are always Gram-positive. Only Gram-negative bacteria produce endotoxin, which is in fact the lipopolysaccharide found in the cell wall.

2. A. F
   B. T
   C. F
   D. F
   E. T

   Viruses are in the size range 0.025–0.2 μm. They can only reproduce in host cells, and do not contain organelles typical of bacteria such as ribosomes or cell walls. Their genetic information is carried on DNA or RNA which may be single- or double-stranded.

3. A. T
    B. F
    C. T
    D. T
    E. F

Staphylococcus aureus is a non-motile, Gram-positive coccus forming grape-like clusters. Some strains can cause food poisoning by production of an enterotoxin.

4. A. T
    B. T
    C. T
    D. F
    E. F

Exotoxins are powerful enzymes found in mainly Gram-positive bacteria. Some can be converted to toxoids, which retain antigenicity but lose toxicity (useful in vaccines, e.g. tetanus). They are high-molecular weight proteins and are thus destroyed by heat. Lipopolysaccharide is endotoxin, not exotoxin.

5. A. T
    B. T
    C. T
    D. T
    E. F

Plasmids can be transferred between bacteria by conjugation or transduction. Since they are intracellular, they cannot possess flagella, which are on the outside of the cell wall.

6. A. F
   B. F
   C. T
   D. T
   E. T

   Clostridium perfringens is a strictly anaerobic Gram-positive
   bacillus that produces spores. In humans it can cause gas
   gangrene by virtue of producing powerful exotoxins, the most
   important being alpha toxin, or phospholipase, and food
   poisoning by producing an enterotoxin that is part of the spore
   coat.

7. A. T
   B. F
   C. T
   D. F
   E. F

   Bacillus cereus produces two enterotoxins, one of which causes
   diarrhoea and abdominal pain, the other causing vomiting. It
   is particularly associated with rice dishes. *Vibrio parahaemolyticus*
   is associated with food poisoning from raw or poorly cooked
   seafood. Its pathogenetic mechanism is not clear.

8. A. T
   B. F
   C. T
   D. F
   E. F

   Ampicillin, like other penicillins, has a mode of action which
   involves interfering with the normal formation of new cell wall.
   It is readily inactivated by many β-lactamase enzymes such as
   those found commonly in staphylococci and *Escherichia coli*.
   Ampicillin is a bactericidal antibiotic itself and does not usually
   interfere with the action of other bactericidal agents; in fact
   there may be synergy, as with ampicillin plus an
   aminoglycoside.

9. A. F
    B. T
    C. F
    D. F
    E. T

Streptococcus pyogenes is another name for the Lancefield Group
A β-haemolytic streptococcus, which, like all streptococci, is
Gram-positive. It is the most common bacterial cause of acute
tonsillitis. Rheumatic fever is thought to be an autoimmune
disease due to the cross-reaction of streptococcal antigens with
cardiac tissue. Actual organisms are not found in the heart
valves. *S. pyogenes* strains remain fully sensitive to penicillin.

10. A. T
    B. F
    C. T
    D. T
    E. F

Aminoglycosides like gentamicin, macrolides like
erythromycin, and chloramphenicol all inhibit protein
synthesis. Penicillin inhibits cell wall formation, while the
quinolone ciprofloxacin inhibits the enzyme DNA gyrase.

11. A. F
    B. T
    C. T
    D. F
    E. T

Some viruses possess enzymes such as DNA or RNA polymerase
in the core. Reverse transcriptase is an RNA-dependent DNA
polymerase characteristic of retroviruses. Haemagglutinin and
neuraminidase project from the lipid envelope of influenza
viruses.

12. A. F
     B. T
     C. F
     D. T
     E. T

Endotoxin is found in the cell wall component lipopolysaccharide in Gram-negative bacteria. One of its biological effects is to stimulate macrophages to release endogenous pyrogens, as part of a cascade of events leading to septic shock. Endotoxin is not responsible for food poisoning (do not confuse with enterotoxin!).

13. A. F
     B. T
     C. T
     D. T
     E. F

Sterility is defined as freedom from all viable forms of microorganisms. It is an absolute state; there are no degrees of sterility. Moist or dry heat, and ethylene oxide gas, under the right conditions, will kill all forms of microbial life including spores. Hypochlorite and ethyl alcohol are disinfectants which kill vegetative cells but not spores.

14. A. T
     B. T
     C. F
     D. T
     E. T

The penicillins, cephalosporins (cefuroxime is one of these), vancomycin and bacitracin all work by inhibiting cell wall synthesis. Trimethoprim acts in the metabolic pathway leading to amino acid, purine and pyrimidine synthesis.

15.　A.　F
　　　B.　F
　　　C.　T
　　　D.　F
　　　E.　T

RSV is the major cause of bronchiolitis in infants and children. It does not cause meningitis. It belongs to the genus *Pneumovirus*, and has a genome of single-stranded RNA.

16.　A.　T
　　　B.　F
　　　C.　T
　　　D.　F
　　　E.　T

The Mantoux test is a skin test for hypersensitivity to tuberculin. The PPD is injected intradermally, and a positive reaction, shown by an inflamed, indurated lesion, is found in people with tuberculosis. The test does not become positive during the first 3–7 weeks after infection. The Tine test is an alternative to the Mantoux test, but is less sensitive.

17.　A.　F
　　　B.　T
　　　C.　T
　　　D.　F
　　　E.　T

Pseudomonas aeruginosa is a Gram-negative bacillus. It produces the pigments pyocyanin and pyoverdin which give a green colour on culture. It is usually sensitive to gentamicin and ceftazidime, but not to amoxycillin. It often causes chronic lung infection in cystic fibrosis patients, and may infect severe burns, sometimes leading to septicaemia.

18. A. T
  B. T
  C. F
  D. T
  E. F

Psittacosis, an atypical pneumonia acquired from infected birds, is caused by *Chlamydia psittaci*. *Chlamydia pneumoniae*, also known as the TWAR agent, is also a cause of atypical pneumonia. *Streptococcus pneumoniae*, the pneumococcus, is the most common cause of community-acquired pneumonia in the UK. *Proteus mirabilis* causes urinary tract infections, and *Mycoplasma hominis* colonizes the genital tract.

19. A. F
  B. T
  C. T
  D. F
  E. F

Escherichia coli is the most common cause of acute cystitis. *Staphylococcus saprophyticus* is an important cause of this condition in sexually active women. The other microorganisms listed would be very rare causes of acute, uncomplicated cystitis.

20. A. F
  B. F
  C. T
  D. F
  E. T

Blood cultures are positive in about 80% of cases. The mortality rate remains 15–30% even in the era of modern antibiotics. Viridans streptococci cause 50–60% of cases. Penicillin plus gentamicin is more appropriate for streptococci than flucloxacillin. Fever is the most commonly found sign.

21. A. T
     B. F
     C. F
     D. T
     E. T

The pneumococcus produces α-haemolysis on blood agar. It is not motile. The optochin test is commonly used to identify it. The polysaccharide capsule prevents binding of antibody to the cell wall of the pneumococcus, thus inhibiting phagocytosis.

22. A. F
     B. F
     C. T
     D. T
     E. T

Pseudomembranous colitis is associated with previous antibiotic therapy and causes diarrhoea. The organism responsible is *Clostridium difficile,* which produces two toxins. One, or both, of these toxins can be detected in the stool. Oral vancomycin is an effective treatment for the condition.

23. A. T
     B. F
     C. T
     D. T
     E. F

The only common causes of acute meningitis in children are *Streptococcus pneumoniae, Haemophilus influenzae* and *Neisseria meningitidis.* Group B β-haemolytic streptococcus causes meningitis in neonates.

24. A. F
     B. T
     C. F
     D. T
     E. F

In the first week of typhoid fever, *Salmonella typhi* causes a septicaemia, thus blood cultures are frequently positive. By the second week, the organism localizes in Peyer's patches of the small intestine and diarrhoea commences. The incubation period is 10–14 days. Man is the only known host of *S. typhi*.

25. A. T
     B. F
     C. T
     D. T
     E. T

Legionella pneumophila, the usual cause of legionnaires' disease, is found widely in the aqueous environment, and is a cause of community-acquired pneumonia. It is usually transmitted to humans in aerosols. Person-to-person spread is unknown. Special media are needed for its laboratory isolation. Erythromycin is usually an effective treatment.

26. A. T
     B. F
     C. T
     D. F
     E. T

Mycobacterium tuberculosis is spread by the droplet nuclei that form in the air after an infected patient coughs or sneezes. *Giardia lamblia* is usually spread in water or food, and *Salmonella typhimurium* in food. Human immunodeficiency virus (HIV) is not spread by aerosol but by blood or other body fluids. *Leptospira icterohaemorrhagiae*, the cause of Weil's disease, usually reaches humans in water contaminated with rats' urine.

27. A. F
B. F
C. T
D. T
E. T

Hepatitis A has an incubation period of 2–6 weeks. A carrier state does not occur. The virus is spread by the faecal–oral route, and often occurs in epidemics. Shellfish from sea water contaminated by sewage can harbour the virus.

28. A. F
B. F
C. F
D. T
E. T

Gentamicin has no useful, clinical activity against streptococci, including *Enterococcus faecalis*, or anaerobes, like *Bacteroides fragilis*.

29. A. T
B. F
C. F
D. T
E. T

Trimethoprim is theoretically teratogenic, being a folate antagonist. Tetracycline crosses the placenta and can bind to fetal bone.

30. A. F
B. T
C. T
D. F
E. T

Salmonella typhi, a cause of enteric fever, is transmitted by contaminated food or water. Good nursing practice and a high standard of hygiene will prevent person-to-person spread by direct contact. Urinary tract infection in patients with long-term catheters cannot be prevented by antibiotics, which are likely merely to lead to infection with resistant organisms.

31. A. T
B. F
C. T
D. F
E. T

The rash of scarlet fever is caused by the erythrogenic toxin of *Streptococcus pyogenes*. Toxic shock syndrome is caused by strains of *Staphylococcus aureus* that produce a particular toxin TSST-1. Scalded skin syndrome results from two other toxins of some strains of *S. aureus*: exfoliative toxins A and B.

32. A. F
B. F
C. F
D. T
E. T

Glutaraldehyde, ethylene oxide and phenol are all too toxic to apply to the skin.

33. A. T
B. F
C. T
D. T
E. F

Haemophilus influenzae requires both X (haemin) and V (NAD) factors. The satellite phenomenon is where colonies of *H. influenzae* grow to a larger size around colonies of staphylococci, which are producing NAD. Encapsulated strains are typed a to f; type b causes most of the invasive infections like meningitis and epiglottitis. Influenza is caused by the influenza virus.

34. A. F
   B. F
   C. F
   D. T
   E. T

Endospores are highly heat resistant. Pili are organs of adhesion and conjugation. Ribosomes are involved in protein synthesis. Peptidoglycan is composed of two alternating sugars: *N*-acetylmuramic acid and *N*-acetyl-glucosamine. Porins are protein channels located in the outer membrane.

35. A. F
   B. T
   C. F
   D. T
   E. T

Falciparum malaria does not relapse after successful treatment. Vivax, ovale and malariae malaria can relapse because of their exo-erythrocytic liver cycle, and hence need a course of primaquine, or similar drug, to prevent relapse. Antimalarial prophylaxis needs to be taken for the whole time in the malarious area and for 4–6 weeks afterwards.

36. A. F
   B. F
   C. F
   D. T
   E. T

Chlamydiae, unlike rickettsiae, do not contain peptidoglycan in their cell walls. They exist in two forms: the elementary body, which is the extracellular and infectious form, and the intracellular reticulate body. Q fever is caused by *Coxiella burnetti*. Chlamydiae do cause pelvic inflammatory disease, and are sensitive to tetracycline.

37.   A.   F
   B.   T
   C.   F
   D.   T
   E.   F

Bubonic plague, caused by *Yersinia pestis*, is transmitted by fleas. Lyme disease, caused by *Borrelia burgdorferi*, is transmitted by ticks. Epidemic typhus is caused by *Rickettsia prowazekii* and is transmitted by lice, usually in times of war or famine.

38.   A.   F
   B.   T
   C.   F
   D.   T
   E.   T

Endotoxin is only found in Gram-negative bacteria. *Clostridium perfringens* is Gram-positive. Phospholipase (alpha toxin) is found in *C. perfringens*. Verotoxin is found in enterohaemorrhagic strains of *Escherichia coli*. *Bacillus cereus* has two types of enterotoxin which can produce food poisoning.

39.   A.   F
   B.   T
   C.   F
   D.   T
   E.   T

Mycobacterium tuberculosis cells divide every 18–24 hours. Colonies are non-pigmented. Pyrazinamide is one of the first-line drugs, together with izoniazid and rifampicin, for treating tuberculosis.

40. A. T
    B. T
    C. F
    D. F
    E. T

Fluconazole belongs to the imidazole class of antifungal agents. Griseofulvin is active against dermatophytes (ringworm fungi) but not yeasts, like *Candida* spp. Metronidazole is not active against fungi.

41. A. T
    B. F
    C. F
    D. F
    E. F

The test for immunity to diphtheria is the Schick test. The usual culture medium for *Corynebacterium diphtheriae* contains tellurite. The genes for toxin production are carried on a bacteriophage. Strains not harbouring the phage are non-toxigenic. Diphtheria vaccine is a toxoid (altered toxin).

42. A. F
    B. F
    C. T
    D. T
    E. T

Haemophilus influenzae and *Neisseria meningitidis* are major causes of meningitis in children, but are very rare in the neonatal period. *Escherichia coli* and group B streptococci are the most common causes of neonatal meningitis. *Listeria* is an uncommon but recognized cause.

43. A. T
    B. F
    C. F
    D. T
    E. T

Penicillin is neurotoxic in very high doses, and can cause fits. Gentamicin is primarily ototoxic and nephrotoxic. The major concern with chloramphenicol is aplastic anaemia. Tetracycline binds to growing bone, causing tooth discoloration, and is therefore contraindicated in children up to 12 years of age.

44. A. F
    B. T
    C. T
    D. F
    E. T

A predominantly lymphocytic response is characteristic of a viral meningitis. Turbidity (due to a high cell count) and high protein are typical of acute bacterial meningitis, as is the finding of bacterial antigen. Glucose is usually below 2.2 mmol/l in bacterial meningitis.

45. A. T
    B. T
    C. F
    D. T
    E. T

The promotor is not a gene but a sequence of nucleotides which is the site for the binding of RNA polymerase, needed for transcription of structural genes.

46. A. T
　　　B. T
　　　C. F
　　　D. F
　　　E. T

Clostridium tetani is a motile, Gram-positive rod with terminal spores, giving a tennis-racket appearance. The Nagler test is for the lecithinase produced by *Clostridium perfringens.* Tetanospasmin, the toxin of *C. tetani*, does prevent the release of inhibitory mediators of motor neurones, thus producing spastic paralysis.

47. A. F
　　　B. T
　　　C. T
　　　D. F
　　　E. T

Spirochetes, including *Treponema pallidum*, are motile by means of axial filaments. A hard chancre is typical of primary syphilis. The Venereal Disease Reference Laboratory (VDRL) test detects reagin, a non-specific, non-treponemal antibody produced in patients with syphilis.

48. A. F
　　　B. T
　　　C. F
　　　D. T
　　　E. F

Temperate phage enters into lysogeny with the host cell. The cleared areas on lawned agar are called plaques. Transduction, not conjugation, is mediated by phage.

49. A. T
   B. T
   C. F
   D. F
   E. T

Sporangiospores are asexual spores, produced within a specialized sac called a sporangium. Conidia are also asexual spores produced on specialized stalks called conidiophores.

50. A. F
   B. T
   C. T
   D. F
   E. T

Neisseria gonorrhoeae is a Gram-negative diplococcus that ferments glucose but not maltose. New York City medium is a widely used selective medium for culturing gonococci. The oxidase test is positive with *Neisseria*. Some strains of gonococci are penicillin-resistant by production of β-lactamase.

51. A. F
   B. T
   C. T
   D. F
   E. F

Streptococcus pyogenes is the Lancefield group A β-haemolytic streptococcus. β-Haemolysis is complete haemolysis of red cells, and is caused by the oxygen-stable haemolysin S. A useful identification test for *S. pyogenes* is its sensitivity to bacitracin.

52. A. F
  B. F
  C. T
  D. T
  E. T

The Gram stain was invented by Christian Gram. The acid-fast stain is so-called because the dye cannot be washed out of the bacterium (i.e. is fast) by acid. Salvarsan was an arsenical compound effective against syphilis. Waksman investigated soil microorganisms and this led to the discovery of streptomycin.

53. A. F
  B. T
  C. T
  D. F
  E. T

Both the nuclear membrane and nucleolus are found in eukaryotes but not in prokaryotes. Ribosomes are found in both.

54. A. F
  B. T
  C. F
  D. T
  E. F

Siderophores are low-molecular weight iron-binding compounds that help remove iron from host tissues, so that it becomes available to the bacterium. Siderophore production is regulated by the amount of iron in the immediate environment.

55. A. T
   B. T
   C. F
   D. T
   E. T

Mucosal surfaces may be protected by secretory immunoglobulin A (IgA), a normal flora of microorganisms (microflora), hydrophilic glycoproteins called mucins that coat the surface, and enzymes such as lysozyme. Exotoxins are toxins produced by some Gram-positive bacteria.

56. A. F
   B. T
   C. F
   D. T
   E. F

The mosquito is a biological vector in the transmission of malaria; the malaria parasite undergoes development and multiplication in the vector. 'Endemic' means a constant, or expected, number of cases in a population. 'Fomites' is a term for inanimate objects (e.g. bedclothes, hospital equipment) which may be involved in indirect transmission.

57. A. T
   B. F
   C. T
   D. F
   E. F

Members of the *Neisseria* genus produce cytochrome oxidase, which is detected by the oxidase test. Immunoglobulin A (IgA) protease inactivates secretory IgA which can block the attachment of organism to host cell. Lecithinase, streptokinase and hyaluronidase are produced by *Clostridium perfringens, Streptococcus pyogenes* and *Strep. pyogenes*, respectively.

58. A. T
   B. F
   C. T
   D. F
   E. F

The 'medusa head' colony is typical of *Bacillus anthracis*, whose exotoxin consists of oedema factor, protective antigen and lethal factor. Anthrax is primarily a disease of herbivorous animals: sheep, cattle and horses. The spores are only produced outside the animal host tissues.

59. A. F
   B. T
   C. F
   D. T
   E. T

Cryptosporidium parvum causes a self-limiting profuse, watery diarrhoea in otherwise normal people; in patients with AIDS it may be fatal. *Giardia lamblia* is a cause of a spectrum of disease varying from acute watery diarrhoea and abdominal cramps to the malabsorption syndrome. *Entamoeba coli* is a non-pathogenic colonizer of the human alimentary tract. *Toxoplasma gondii* is a parasite primarily of cats, but occasionally infects humans causing a glandular fever-like illness, or congenital infection in newborn babies. *Entamoeba histolytica* is the cause of amoebic dysentery.

60. A. F
   B. T
   C. F
   D. T
   E. T

In the early stages of human immunodeficiency virus (HIV) infection, the T4 cell count is normal. The usual HIV tests detect anti-HIV antibodies. HIV belongs to a class of retrovirus called human T-lymphotropic viruses (HTLV). (ELISA is the acronym for enzyme-linked immunosorbent assay.)

61. A. F
  B. T
  C. T
  D. F
  E. T

Listeria monocytogenes is a short Gram-positive rod, which produces a narrow zone of β-haemolysis on blood agar. It is a recognized cause of meningitis, particularly in newborn infants and in the immunocompromised. It has been isolated from certain soft cheeses.

62. A. F
  B. T
  C. F
  D. T
  E. F

Vibrio cholerae is a Gram-negative curved rod, motile by means of a polar flagellum. Thiosulphate citrate bile salt sucrose (TCBS) agar is a selective medium often used to culture *V. cholerae*. Non-01 strains can cause gastroenteritis and produce a cholera-like toxin. Cholera enterotoxin affects adenyl cyclase, ultimately leading to an efflux of water from mucosal surfaces and hence watery diarrhoea. The major causes of death in cholera are shock, metabolic acidosis and renal failure.

63. A. T
  B. T
  C. F
  D. F
  E. T

L-Forms can revert back to the parental form, whereas mycoplasmas do not revert to any other form. Mycoplasma cell membranes are reinforced with sterols. Penicillin has no effect on mycoplasmas. A characteristic of *Ureaplasma urealyticum* is that it hydrolyses urea. L-Forms have now been found in most species of bacteria.

64. A. T
     B. T
     C. F
     D. F
     E. T

Lymphogranuloma venereum is a sexually transmitted disease caused by *Chlamydia trachomatis*. This organism is also a cause of trachoma and pelvic inflammatory disease. Farmers' lung is a hypersensitivity reaction to thermophilic actinomycetes on mouldy hay. Q fever is caused by *Coxiella burnetti*.

65. A. F
     B. T
     C. T
     D. T
     E. T

Staphylococcus epidermidis often causes infections related to indwelling prosthetic devices. The major causes of neonatal meningitis are *Escherichia coli* and group B streptococci.

66. A. T
     B. F
     C. T
     D. F
     E. F

Acanthamoeba is a free-living soil amoeba which can cause chronic granulomatous amoebic encephalitis. It can also cause keratitis, a serious infection of the cornea, particularly in contact lens wearers.

67. A. F
 B. F
 C. T
 D. T
 E. T

Although rifampicin is regarded as the first choice agent, both ceftriaxone by injection and oral ciprofloxacin are also effective. Penicillin, although a standard treatment for meningococcal meningitis, is ineffective as prophylaxis.

68. A. T
 B. F
 C. T
 D. F
 E. T

Clinical symptoms of pyelonephritis will occur in 30–40% of women with untreated bacteriuria of pregnancy. Ciprofloxacin, and other quinolones, should be avoided in pregnancy because of potential teratogenicity.

69. A. F
 B. T
 C. F
 D. T
 E. F

Gentamicin and vancomycin are potentially toxic agents and require blood level monitoring. Although amphotericin B is also toxic, blood levels are of no help in adjusting the dosage.

70. A. F
 B. T
 C. T
 D. T
 E. F

Bacteroides fragilis is an anaerobic non-sporing Gram-negative bacillus found in the gastrointestinal tract. It is commonly isolated from peritonitis, brain and liver abscesses, but is a very rare cause of endocarditis or meningitis.

71. A. F
B. F
C. T
D. T
E. T

Ciprofloxacin, a quinolone, inhibits DNA gyrase whilst polymixin affects the cell membrane.

72. A. T
B. T
C. T
D. T
E. F

Campylobacter jejuni is a common cause of gastroenteritis, often with cramping abdominal pain and bloody diarrhoea. The usual treatment is erythromycin. In culture, it will grow at 43°C in an atmosphere containing 5% oxygen and 10% CO_2.

73. A. T
B. T
C. F
D. F
E. T

Actinomycosis usually involves the lower jaw, following dental disease or extraction. 'Sulphur granules' are actually macro-colonies of the organism *Actinomyces israelii*, which is a strictly anaerobic, branching bacterium, sensitive to penicillin.

74. A. F
B. F
C. F
D. F
E. T

The transparent tape-slide method is used for diagnosing threadworm infections. The usual pathogen in amoebic dysentery is *Entamoeba histolytica*, motile trophozoites of which can be seen in fresh stools. The usual site of amoebic abscesses is the liver.

75. A. T
　　B. F
　　C. F
　　D. T
　　E. F

Ciprofloxacin and chloramphenicol are recognized treatments for typhoid fever. *Salmonella typhi* is usually very sensitive to them, and they penetrate well into cells. The other agents listed may be active in laboratory tests, but clinically fail, probably because they do not penetrate into cells well enough to kill intracellular *S. typhi*.

Histopathology – Answers

76. A. T
B. F
C. F
D. T
E. T

Apoptosis or programmed cell death is an energy-dependent process which involves activation of cellular non-lysosomal endonucleases. The cytopathic effect of most viruses does not involve integration into host DNA. Indeed, in many viral infections cell death is immunologically mediated, a process involving cytotoxic T lymphocytes recognizing viral proteins expressed at the surface of infected cells. During the process of irreversible cell injury due to ischaemia there is a dramatic *increase* in the levels of cytosolic calcium because of decreased activity of membrane ATP-ases. In immune-mediated injuries, perforans and granzymes released by cytotoxic T lymphocytes lead to lysis of cell membranes. Loss of selective membrane permeability is an essential feature of cell death or necrosis.

77. A. F
B. F
C. T
D. T
E. T

Fibrinoid necrosis occurs only in the walls of blood vessels in conditions such as malignant phase hypertension and some vasculitides. Necrosis in renal infarction is generally of coagulative type. Necrosis can be identified by the presence of karyolysis, karyorrhexis and pyknosis; these changes are due to progressive degradation of nuclear components. Necrosis normally leads to acute inflammation within a tissue and may be associated with dystrophic calcification – a process in which calcium salts are deposited in tissues although the serum levels of calcium and phosphate are within the normal range.

78. A. F
B. T
C. F
D. T
E. F

Although haemochromatosis is predominantly seen in males, it is inherited as an autosomal recessive trait. Red/green colour blindness is the commonest X-linked condition affecting almost 1 in 10 males. Adrenogenital syndrome is an inherited disorder which is transmitted as an autosomal recessive trait. Duchenne muscular dystrophy is an X-linked condition but myotonic dystrophy is an autosomal dominant disorder.

79. A. F
B. T
C. F
D. T
E. T

A response of many tissues to increased functional demand is an increase in organ size. When this occurs through an increase in cell number, it is referred to as *hyperplasia* but when it is due to increase in cell size without replication it is *hypertrophy*. In the myocardium, the cells are permanent (i.e. they are incapable of further division); enlargement of the left ventricle when there is obstruction to outflow is due to hypertrophy. Gynaecomastia is pathological breast hyperplasia in males and occurs around puberty and in conditions associated with high oestrogen levels such as cirrhosis. The transformation of one type of differentiated tissue into another, such as occurs in bronchi in response to chronic irritation due to cigarette smoke, is referred to as *metaplasia*. Diabetic retinopathy is a pathological form of hyperplasia where there is growth of capillaries in the retina. Chronic hypoxia leads to a 'physiological' hyperplasia of erythrocyte precursors and a subsequent increase in the number of circulating red blood cells.

80. A. F
      B. F
      C. T
      D. T
      E. F

Platelet-activating factor and plasminogen activator inhibitors are prothrombotic. The main plasminogen activator inhibitor produced by endothelial cells (PAI-1) inhibits the production of plasmin and hence decreases turnover of fibrin. Thrombomodulin is an anticoagulant and prostacyclin prevents platelet aggregation. Endothelin-1 is an important vasoactive molecule produced by endothelial cells; it mediates vasoconstriction but is not directly involved in haemostasis.

81. A. T
      B. F
      C. T
      D. T
      E. T

Disseminated intravascular coagulation (DIC) occurs when there is massive or prolonged release of thromboplastins from damaged endothelial cells or when there is release of other soluble tissue factors which can activate the coagulation system. In septicaemia and in tissue trauma (e.g. burns) there is endothelial damage and this may lead to DIC. In amniotic fluid embolism, tissue factor (factor III) is released into the maternal circulation triggering coagulation. Many tumours, in particular mucin-secreting carcinomas, release procoagulant substances and can be complicated by DIC. Von Willebrand's disease is an inherited deficiency of von Willebrand factor (factor VIII-related antigen); this leads to a bleeding diathesis but is not associated with intravascular coagulation.

82. A. F
    B. T
    C. T
    D. F
    E. T

In contrast to other forms of shock (e.g. hypovolaemic, cardiogenic), in endotoxic shock there is peripheral vasodilatation. This is generally associated with a normal (or even increased) cardiac output. A number of soluble mediators released by endothelial cells and macrophages are involved in producing the haemodynamic effects; tumour necrosis factor α plays a crucial role. In common with other forms of shock, decreased tissue perfusion leads to hypoxic injury and in turn this produces a metabolic acidosis. Endotoxic shock is a serious condition with a high mortality rate.

83. A. T
    B. F
    C. T
    D. T
    E. F

Histamine is the best-known endogenous mediator of acute inflammation. It mediates the immediate transient phase of increased vascular permeability in acute inflammatory responses. By-products of complement activation, in particular C5a and C3a, are also involved in bringing about increased vascular permeability and this is mediated (at least in part) by their ability to stimulate histamine release from mast cells. Leukotrienes are derivatives of arachadonic acid and these can also increase vascular permeability. Interleukin-6 is a mediator of the acute phase response but has no direct action on endothelium. Interleukin-8 is a chemokine which is involved in recruitment of neutrophils in acute inflammation but has no effects on permeability.

84. A. F
   B. T
   C. T
   D. T
   E. T

The classic pathway of complement is activated principally by antigen–antibody complexes. Cobra venom activates the alternative pathway of complement as do endotoxins. The final common product of classic and alternative pathways is the membrane attack complex C5b6789, which can mediate cell lysis. C1 inhibitor is one of three control enzymes that regulate the activity of the classic pathway; inherited deficiency of C1 inhibitor leads to hereditary angio-oedema. Complement can be activated by products of kinin, coagulation and fibrinolytic systems.

85. A. F
   B. T
   C. T
   D. F
   E. T

Staphylococcus aureus classically produces pyogenic inflammation. Exposure to beryllium provokes granulomatous lesions in the lungs which may lead to fibrosis. Widespread granulomatous inflammation occurs in immunosuppressed patients infected with *Mycobacterium avium intracellulare*; this is frequently encountered in acquired immune deficiency syndrome (AIDS). Measles virus can produce a giant cell pneumonia but in this condition the giant cells are formed by fusion of infected epithelial cells and this is not associated with granuloma formation. Sarcoidosis is a systemic granulomatous condition of uncertain aetiology.

86. A. F
    B. F
    C. T
    D. T
    E. F

In industrialized nations, the most common cause of vitamin A deficiency is malabsorption as a result of hepatobiliary or pancreatic dysfunction; it is not a feature of chronic renal failure. Vitamin A deficiency has no effect on blood clotting although another fat-soluble vitamin, vitamin K, is required for the synthesis of four clotting factors in the liver. One of the most serious consequences of vitamin A deficiency is xerophthalmia which may lead to corneal ulceration and blindness. Hypervitaminosis A has been associated with several forms of liver injury including cirrhosis. There is no evidence that excess vitamin A is carcinogenic. Indeed, it may induce regression in some premalignant lesions.

87. A. F
    B. F
    C. T
    D. T
    E. F

The first matrix proteins to be laid down in granulation tissue are fibronectin and proteoglycans. This is followed by type III collagen and later type I collagen. The process of angiogenesis or neovascularization is characterized by proliferation of vessels at right angles to the wound surface. Fibroblast activity is controlled by several growth factors; transforming growth factor (TGF) β is the most important in stimulating collagen synthesis. Myofibroblasts in granulation tissue have contractile properties which are thought to be important in wound healing. Epithelioid macrophages are found in granulomas but *not* in granulation tissue.

88. A. F
    B. T
    C. T
    D. T
    E. F

Although vitamin D deficiency may impair the healing of fractures, it does not have any effect on skin wound healing (vitamin C deficiency or scurvy may interfere with wound healing as it acts as a co-factor in collagen synthesis). Diabetes mellitus and Cushing's syndrome are two systemic disorders known to impair healing while poor blood supply is an example of a local factor. Magnesium deficiency has no effect on wound healing.

89. A. T
    B. F
    C. T
    D. T
    E. F

Type II hypersensitivity reactions (antibody-dependent cytotoxicity) usually involve antibodies of immunoglobulin (Ig) G or IgM classes. Autoimmune thrombocytopaenic purpura is caused by an autoantibody which reacts with a surface protein of platelets. Rhesus (Rh) incompatibility is also an example of type II hypersensitivity. It occurs in rhesus D +ve children born to rhesus D −ve mothers who have been previously sensitized to RhD in earlier pregnancies. The Mantoux reaction is an example of cell-mediated immunity (type IV hypersensitivity).

90. A. T
    B. F
    C. F
    D. T
    E. T

Addison's disease is an autoimmune disorder leading to adrenal gland hypofunction. By contrast, Conn's syndrome is adrenal cortical hyperfunction with excess production of mineralocorticoids by a benign adrenal tumour. Although the effects of rheumatoid arthritis are most clearly manifest in joints, this is a systemic immune complex disease with protean extra-articular manifestations. Myaesthenia gravis is an autoimmune disease affecting skeletal muscle mediated by anti-acetylcholine receptor antibodies. Type 1 diabetes mellitus is another organ-specific autoimmune disease where there is selective destruction of β cells in pancreatic islets.

91. A. F
  B. F
  C. T
  D. T
  E. T

Amyloid is an insoluble mixture of proteins arranged as antiparallel β pleated sheets. In primary amyloidosis the predominant proteins are immunoglobulin light chains and it is therefore of AL type. This is also the form of amyloid found in multiple myeloma. Amyloid of AH type (β_2 microglobulin) occurs in patients with chronic renal failure on haemodialysis; this form of amyloidosis predominantly affects joints. Systemic amyloidosis commonly affects the heart leading to a congestive cardiomyopathy with cardiac failure.

92. A. F
  B. T
  C. T
  D. F
  E. F

Wilson's disease is an autosomal recessive condition associated with excess copper storage. Iron overload can lead to congestive cardiomyopathy and cardiac failure. Increased tissue deposition of iron is seen in thalassaemia where there is ineffective erythropoiesis and marrow hyperplasia. In iron overload, iron is deposited in endocrine organs and this leads to hypofunction; pituitary failure may occur and this can be associated with impaired adrenal cortical function. Genetic haemochromatosis is seen more frequently in males and this is due in part to the protective effect of menstrual blood loss in females.

93. A. F
     B. T
     C. F
     D. T
     E. T

DNA synthesis occurs only during S phase. Cells enter G_1 phase from G_0 under the influence of signal peptides known as competence factors. M phase (mitosis) is the shortest part of the cell cycle lasting less than one hour. Transition from G_2 to M requires phosphokinases, in particular mitosis promoting factor (MPF). G_0 phase is the stage of growth arrest from which cells can be activated to enter the cell cycle.

94. A. F
     B. T
     C. T
     D. F
     E. T

Seminoma is a malignant tumour of the testis which frequently metastasizes. Leiomyoma is a benign tumour of smooth muscle cells. Squamous papillomas are benign tumours most frequently seen on the skin. Glioblastoma multiforme is a highly malignant brain tumour. Neurofibroma is a benign tumour of neural origin.

95. A. T
     B. T
     C. F
     D. F
     E. T

Carcinoembryonic antigen (CEA) is present in many bowel carcinomas; although it is not a tumour-specific product, serum levels are used to monitor tumour recurrence. Thyroglobulin can be used to detect the presence of metastatic tumours in patients who have been treated for thyroid carcinoma by thyroidectomy. Tumour necrosis factor α is a cytokine whose principal activity is in inflammatory processes; it is *not* used as a tumour marker. C reactive protein is an acute phase protein. βHCG (human chorionic gonadotrophin) is a marker for trophoblastic tumours.

96. A. T
    B. T
    C. F
    D. T
    E. T

Nasopharyngeal carcinoma and Hodgkin's disease have both been associated with Epstein–Barr virus. There is no evidence that viruses play a role in the development of colorectal tumours. There is a strong association between infection with hepatitis B and hepatitis C viruses and the development of hepatocellular carcinoma. Cancer of the cervix has been associated with herpes simplex virus and human papilloma virus.

97. A. F
    B. T
    C. F
    D. T
    E. T

Cadherins mediate cell–cell adhesion and these molecules are often down-regulated in malignant tumours. Integrin molecules mediate cell–matrix interactions and expression of these proteins is often altered in tumours showing an aggressive growth pattern. Production of matrix metalloproteinases such as collagenases by tumour cells is thought to be crucial for invasion through basement membranes. Malignant tumours frequently show up-regulation of growth factor receptors and the cells may themselves produce peptides which act as autocrine growth factors. Invasion is enhanced by the production of new vessels around tumours and this is mediated by the production of angiogenesis factors released by malignant cells.

98. A. F
     B. F
     C. T
     D. T
     E. T

Asbestos exposure is associated with development of bronchial and pleural tumours. Benzo(*a*)pyrene is a potent carcinogen present in tobacco smoke which is implicated in carcinoma of bronchus. Exposure of vinyl chloride monomer in the plastics industry is strongly associated with the development of liver angiosarcomas. Aflatoxins are found in mouldy nuts and cereals and have been implicated in liver carcinogenesis, as have nitrosamines found in some foodstuffs.

99. A. F
     B. F
     C. T
     D. T
     E. F

Tumour suppressor genes are genes whose expression appears to inhibit neoplastic transformation. Tumorigenesis can be associated with inactivation of these genes. p53 and RB-1 are both tumour suppressor genes while c-*myc*, h-*ras* and *bcl2* are all cellular protooncogenes. c-*myc* is involved in control of the cell cycle. The *ras* genes are involved in signal transduction and control a number of cellular functions. *bcl2* is a so-called anti-apoptosis gene.

100. A. T
      B. T
      C. F
      D. T
      E. T

Some tumours, most notably small cell lung cancers, inappropriately secrete adrenocorticotrophic hormone (ACTH) and this can lead to Cushing's syndrome. Hypercalcaemia of malignancy is partly caused by bone erosion by metastatic tumours but some primary tumours secrete parathormone-like substances which can lead to increased bone turnover and hypercalcaemia. Iron deficiency anaemia in malignancy is most often caused by direct effects of tumours with chronic blood loss (e.g. gastrointestinal tumours). Dermatomyositis is a vasculitic condition involving skin and muscle and is a non-metastatic complication of several tumours as is acanthosis nigricans where there is increased melanin deposition in the axillae and groin.

101. A. F
       B. T
       C. F
       D. F
       E. T

Dystrophic calcification is a deposition of calcium salts in tissues when there are normal circulating calcium levels. By contrast, metastatic calcification occurs when there is a systemic disorder with hypercalcaemia. Primary hyperparathyroidism, bony metastases and sarcoidosis are all associated with hypercalcaemia and therefore lead to metastatic calcification whereas calcification found in atheroma and in fat necrosis is dystrophic.

102. A. T
       B. F
       C. F
       D. T
       E. F

Diabetes mellitus and systemic hypertension are both known to predispose to the development of atheroma. High density lipoprotein (HDL) can be regarded as a 'protective' lipid fraction; several studies have shown that there is an inverse relationship between HDL levels and the risk of atheroma. Atheroma is more likely to develop in individuals showing type A behavioural pattern. Anaemia may exacerbate the effects of atheroma (e.g. cardiac failure) but there is no evidence that anaemia *per se* predisposes to the development of atheroma.

103. A. T
B. T
C. F
D. F
E. T

Systemic hypertension is frequently seen in chronic glomerulonephritis; renal diseases represent the most common causes of secondary hypertension. Phaeochromocytomas are tumours of the adrenal medulla and secrete adrenaline or noradrenaline; these may lead to malignant phase hypertension. Cirrhosis is associated with hypertension in the portal venous system but not with systemic hypertension. Klinefelter's syndrome is a chromosomal abnormality in which there is an extra X chromosome; there are no associations between this condition and systemic hypertension. In Conn's syndrome (primary hyperaldosteronism) there is elevated circulating aldosterone and this stimulates sodium and water retention causing hypertension.

104. A. T
B. T
C. F
D. F
E. T

Wegener's granulomatosis is a systemic vasculitis which is associated with necrotizing granulomatous inflammation that affects the respiratory tract and the kidneys. Henoch–Schönlein purpura is characterized by vasculitis involving small vessels in the skin, gastrointestinal tract and kidneys; it is most commonly seen in children. Senile purpura, by contrast, is seen in elderly individuals and is caused by deficient collagen formation around dermal blood vessels. Dermatitis herpetiformis is a bullous condition of the skin which is associated with coeliac disease; vasculitis is not a feature of this condition. Buerger's disease (thromboangiitis obliterans) is a vasculitis of medium-sized and small arteries and veins which occurs predominantly in males and which is associated with cigarette smoking.

105. A. T
　　　B. F
　　　C. T
　　　D. F
　　　E. F

Syphilitic aneurysms classically occur in the arch of the aorta; these are now rare. Thoracic aortic aneurysms can cause recurrent laryngeal palsy by compression. Atheromatous aneurysms in the abdominal aorta are most frequently seen below the level of the renal artery. They are more commonly seen in males than in females. Arteriovenous aneurysms and racemose aneurysms occurring in relation to trauma can rarely be associated with high output cardiac failure but aortic aneurysms are not associated with this complication.

106. A. F
　　　B. T
　　　C. F
　　　D. T
　　　E. T

Recurrent pulmonary thromboembolism gives rise to pulmonary hypertension and *right* ventricular hypertrophy. Renal artery stenosis is associated with the development of systemic hypertension which in turn can lead to left ventricular hypertrophy. Tricuspid valve disease is associated with right ventricular hypertrophy. Coarctation of the aorta leads to pressure overload and left ventricular hypertrophy while aortic valve incompetence leads to increased volume load and left ventricular hypertrophy.

107. A. T
　　　B. F
　　　C. T
　　　D. F
　　　E. T

Polyarteritis nodosa is a rare cause of coronary artery occlusion and myocardial infarction. Alkaline phosphatase levels are not altered following uncomplicated myocardial infarction. Dressler's syndrome is characterized by pericardial and pleural effusions, fever and leucocytosis, and occurs several weeks after myocardial infarctions. Myocardial infarctions are most commonly seen following occlusion of the anterior descending branch of the left coronary artery. Involvement of papillary muscles in myocardial infarction can lead to their rupture and acute mitral valve incompetence.

108. A. F
     B. F
     C. T
     D. T
     E. T

Takayasu's disease is a fibrosing vasculitis affecting the aorta and large arteries. Giant cell arteritis is another vasculitis which most commonly affects the temporal artery although other vessels can be affected. Coxsackie virus infection is sometimes associated with myocarditis and there is evidence that this may lead in some patients to congestive cardiomyopathy. Toxoplasmosis may lead to myocarditis in neonates and in immunocompromised patients. In acute rheumatic fever there is a pancarditis and in some cases the myocarditis can lead to acute cardiac failure.

109. A. F
     B. T
     C. T
     D. F
     E. T

Rheumatic fever usually follows streptococcal pharyngitis. Aschoff bodies are found in the connective tissue septa of the myocardium and are pathognomonic of rheumatic fever. Several forms of skin rash occur in rheumatic fever and of these the most common is erythema marginatum. Although cardiac failure can occur during the acute illness, myocardial function usually recovers completely. (Recurrent bouts of rheumatic fever can of course lead to rheumatic valve disease and hence chronic heart failure: this is fortunately now rare.) Acute rheumatic fever is mediated in part by antibodies to streptococcal antigens which cross-react with sarcolemmal proteins of cardiac myocytes.

110. A. T
B. F
C. F
D. T
E. T

Fallot's tetralogy is the most common form of cyanotic congenital heart disease. It comprises: (i) right ventricular outflow obstruction, (ii) right ventricular hypertrophy, (iii) interventricular septal defect, and (iv) dextraposition of the aortic root. Patent ductus arteriosus may lead to heart failure but is not normally associated with cyanosis. Coarctation leads to systemic hypertension but patients with this disorder are not cyanotic. In truncus arteriosus the aorta and pulmonary arteries arise from a common vessel and this abnormality leads to cyanosis. Cyanosis is also a feature of transposition of the great vessels where there is failure of the proximal aorta and pulmonary artery to undergo the normal patterns of development and as a consequence the aorta arises from the right ventricle and the pulmonary artery from the left ventricle.

111. A. F
B. T
C. T
D. T
E. F

Although pericarditis is frequently seen in acute renal failure, it is not a feature of hepatic failure. Acute pericarditis occurs in some cases of rheumatoid arthritis and may progress to constrictive pericarditis. Tuberculous pericarditis may complicate pulmonary tuberculosis; this may also lead to constrictive pericarditis. Direct spread of tumour from carcinoma of the bronchus into the pericardium can produce pericarditis. Although pericarditis is seen in some cases of hypothyroidism it is not a feature of hyperthyroidism.

112. A.   F
      B.   F
      C.   T
      D.   T
      E.   T

Emphysema is enlargement of the airspaces distal to the terminal bronchioles (abnormal and permanent dilatation of the bronchi is bronchiectasis). In α_1-antitrypsin deficiency it is usually panacinar emphysema that develops. Focal dust emphysema is seen in coal workers and in this condition the dilated respiratory bronchioles are surrounded by carbon pigment. Interstitial emphysema often follows puncture of the lung surface as a result of trauma; air is expelled into the interlobular septa and into soft tissues of the hilum. Centrilobular emphysema leads to chronic hypoxia and carbon dioxide retention and this frequently leads to right ventricular failure. By contrast, panacinar emphysema less frequently leads to left ventricular failure.

113. A.   F
      B.   T
      C.   T
      D.   T
      E.   F

Klebsiella pneumonia is most frequently seen in elderly debilitated patients. Legionnaires' disease can be associated with either a lobar or a bronchopneumonia. Cytomegalovirus pneumonia is most frequently seen in patients who are immunosuppressed and this is a common complication of transplantation, in particular bone marrow transplantation. Measles produces a giant cell pneumonia in which the giant cells are formed by fusion of alveolar pneumocytes. Pneumococcal lobar pneumonia normally undergoes complete resolution and fibrosis occurs in less than 5% of cases.

114. A. T
B. T
C. F
D. F
E. T

Busulphan is a cytotoxic drug used in cancer chemotherapy which may produce adult respiratory distress sydrome and pulmonary fibrosis. Asbestos exposure can also give rise to diffuse pulmonary fibrosis. Cigarette smoking is associated with chronic bronchitis and emphysema but does not appear to be related to the development of diffuse pulmonary fibrosis. Lymphangitis carcinomatosis is widespread permeation of pulmonary lymphatics by metastatic tumour; this is not associated with fibrosis. In bird fancier's lung exposure to inhaled antigens leads to extrinsic allergic alveolitis and repeated exposure may lead to the development of diffuse interstitial fibrosis.

115. A. T
B. F
C. T
D. T
E. F

Some bronchial carcinomas secrete antidiuretic hormone (ADH) and this can produce the syndrome of inappropriate ADH secretion with consequent hyponatraemia. Overall, the most common histological type is squamous cell carcinoma. Although the most frequent malignant tumour arising in relation to asbestos exposure is mesothelioma, there is an increased risk of carcinoma of the bronchus, particularly when the patient is a smoker. Cushing's syndrome can occur in carcinoma of the bronchus due to secretion of an adrenocorticotrophic hormone (ACTH)-like hormone by the tumour; this is most commonly seen with small cell (oat cell) carcinoma. Most peripheral malignant lung tumours are adenocarcinomas.

116. A. F
   B. F
   C. T
   D. T
   E. F

Malignant tumours of the upper third of the oesophagus are most commonly squamous in type. There are remarkable geographic variations in the incidence of oesophageal carcinoma and the incidence is particularly high in some parts of the Far East such as China. Several environmental agents such as cigarette smoking and alcohol are thought to predispose to the development of carcinoma of the oesophagus. Achalasia is another predisposing factor. Carcinoma of the oesophagus normally causes death by local spread rather than metastatic complications. There may be infiltration to adjacent structures and lymphatic spread to local paraoesophageal lymph nodes is common but haematogenous spread to distant organs is rare.

117. A. F
   B. T
   C. T
   D. T
   E. F

Type B chronic gastritis is caused by *Helicobacter pylori* infection. This organism is also associated with lymphocytic gastritis; in the latter it is thought to be an abnormal response to *Helicobacter* infection. Type A chronic gastritis is an autoimmune condition which leads to vitamin B_{12} malabsorption and the development of megaloblastic anaemia (pernicious anaemia). Gastritis associated with biliary reflux is characterized by foveolar hyperplasia, oedema and vasodilatation in the absence of a significant inflammatory infiltrate. Fungal gastritis is exceptionally rare and occurs only in immunosuppressed individuals.

118. A. T
B. F
C. T
D. F
E. T

Coeliac disease is a common cause of malabsorption. It is characterized by villous atrophy and crypt hyperplasia and is thought to be a result of hypersensitivity to gluten which is present in foodstuffs such as cereals; there is a genetic predisposition to this disease with a strong association with HLA-B8. In coeliac disease there is an increased incidence of small bowel lymphoma which tends to be of T cell type.

119. A. F
B. F
C. T
D. T
E. F

Pseudomembranous colitis is caused by exotoxins produced by the organism *Clostridium difficile.* This is most commonly seen in patients who have been treated with antibiotics such as lincomycin and ampicillin. Granulomas are not a feature of this condition. The diagnosis can be made on the basis of identifying *C. difficile* exotoxins in stool samples. The condition has a high mortality rate but in patients who survive there is resolution of the changes and there is no evidence that there is any increased incidence of tumour.

120. A. F
B. T
C. F
D. F
E. T

Ulcerative colitis is one form of chronic inflammatory bowel disease. It is confined to the large intestine and is most commonly seen in the distal colon although in some cases it may affect the entire colon. There is a strong association with primary sclerosing cholangitis (and cholangiocarcinoma). As it affects only the large bowel it does not lead to malabsorption. (By contrast, this is an important feature of Crohn's disease.)

There are a number of common systemic manifestations of ulcerative colitis and these include ankylosing spondylitis and iridocyclitis.

121. A. T
   B. F
   C. T
   D. F
   E. T

Pancreatic insufficiency is a result of chronic pancreatitis leading to a deficiency of lipases within the small intestine which in turn leads to fat malabsorption. Staphylococcal food poisoning is an acute disorder characterized by vomiting, fever and sometimes diarrhoea but this is not associated with malabsorption. Abetalipoproteinaemia is a rare inherited (autosomal recessive) condition in which there is impaired transport of triglycerides from the enterocytes to the lymphatics of small intestinal villae; this abnormality leads to fat malabsorption. Diverticular disease specifically affects the colon (in particular the left side of colon) and this is not associated with malabsorption. Giardiasis is a protozoal infection of the small intestine which can be associated with malabsorption.

122. A. T
   B. F
   C. F
   D. T
   E. F

Familial adenomatous polyposis is an autosomal dominant condition in which specific abnormalities on chromosome 5 lead to a predisposition to the formation of colonic adenomas and subsequent malignant transformation. Most malignant tumours in the colon are adenocarcinomas. These tumours are *staged* using the Dukes' classification; grading is achieved using cytological parameters (i.e. degree of differentiation). Ulcerative colitis predisposes to the development of colonic carcinoma. Colonic carcinoma is more prevalent in Western countries than in developing nations; this is thought to be related to differences in dietary fibre intake.

123. A. T
    B. F
    C. T
    D. F
    E. T

Chronic alcohol abuse leads to steatohepatitis in approximately 30% of patients; this leads to the development of cirrhosis in approximately one third of these individuals. There is no apparent increase in gall bladder disease in chronic alcoholics. However, acute pancreatitis is a complication of acute alcohol intoxication. Alcohol abuse is associated with a number of disorders of the central nervous system including Wernicke–Korsakoff syndrome and Marchiafava–Bignami syndrome. However, subacute combined degeneration of the spinal cord is not a feature of alcoholism but results from chronic vitamin B_{12} deficiency. Alcohol abuse is a cause of congestive cardiomyopathy.

124. A. F
    B. F
    C. T
    D. F
    E. T

Hepatatis A causes a self-limiting disease with no risk of progression to chronicity. Acute paracetamol intoxication causes liver cell necrosis; the degree of injury is related to the amount of drug ingested – when severe this may be associated with acute liver failure but there is no risk of subsequent development of chronic liver disease. Hepatitis C is now recognized to be one of the principal causes worldwide of cirrhosis. Leptospirosis is caused by a spirochaete transmitted by vermin; infection causes liver cell necrosis and cholestasis but does not lead to chronic liver disease. α_1-Antitrypsin deficiency is one of the inherited abnormalities associated with the development of cirrhosis; this most frequently occurs in individuals who are ZZ homozygotes.

125. A. F
     B. T
     C. F
     D. T
     E. T

Primary biliary cirrhosis is a disorder of intrahepatic bile ducts and is characterized by granulomatous and lymphocytic destruction of bile duct radicles. There is a female : male ratio of approximately 9 : 1 and the disease is associated with a number of other autoimmune conditions including Sjögren's syndrome and scleroderma. Circulating antimitochondrial antibodies are found in over 95% but antinuclear factors are rarely present. As with other forms of chronic cholestasis serum cholesterol levels may be grossly elevated.

126. A. T
     B. F
     C. T
     D. T
     E. T

Reye's syndrome occurs in children and in some is the result of an abnormal response to salicylates; liver biopsies in Reye's syndrome characteristically show small droplet fatty liver (microvesicular steatosis). The classic histological feature of autoimmune chronic hepatitis is piecemeal necrosis; steatosis is not a feature. Large droplet fatty liver (macrovesicular steatosis) is seen in alcoholic liver disease, type 2 diabetes mellitus (and obesity) and in protein energy malnutrition (kwashiorkor).

127. A. F
     B. T
     C. F
     D. F
     E. T

Type 1 diabetes mellitus is the insulin-dependent form which normally presents in childhood. Autoimmune phenomena are described in this condition including the presence of circulating anti-islet cell antibodies. Patients are generally thin; by contrast, type 2 diabetes mellitus is strongly associated with obesity. In type 1 diabetes mellitus there is selective destruction of β cells with preservation of α, δ and PP cells. Atheroma occurs at an earlier age and is more severe in patients with diabetes than in non-diabetic individuals and this leads to an increased risk of ischaemic heart disease.

128. A. T
     B. T
     C. F
     D. T
     E. T

Alcohol abuse and gallstones are the most common causes of acute pancreatitis accounting for over 75% of all cases in the UK. Hypothermia leads to acute pancreatitis principally because of hypotension. Direct trauma can lead to disruption of the gland with release of enzymes and consequent pancreatitis. Cystic fibrosis is associated with a chronic obliterative process in the pancreas which in time leads to pancreatic insufficiency.

129. A. T
     B. F
     C. T
     D. F
     E. T

Granulomatous lymphadenopathy can occur in any generalized granulomatous condition including sarcoidosis and Crohn's disease. Mycobacterial infections represent the most common infective cause of granulomatous lymphadenopathy but toxoplasmosis infection is also a frequent cause. Epstein–Barr virus infection (glandular fever) is associated with paracortical hyperplasia but not with granuloma formation. Lymphadenopathy in rheumatoid arthritis is the result of follicular hyperplasia.

130. A. F
B. T
C. T
D. T
E. F

The most common subtype in the UK is nodular sclerosing which accounts for over two-thirds of cases. Hodgkin's disease can be staged according to the distribution of nodes involved; stage 3 refers to disease which is above and below the diaphragm but in the absence of bone marrow or liver involvement. Lymphocyte predominant and some forms of nodular sclerosing Hodgkin's disease have an excellent prognosis with a five-year survival of over 90%. The Reed–Sternberg cell and its variant forms are considered to be the neoplastic element in Hodgkin's disease; the lymphocytic component is thought to be reactive and is polyclonal.

131. A. T
B. F
C. T
D. T
E. F

Low grade T cell lymphomas can present as skin lesions known as mycosis fungoides; when this is associated with the presence of tumour cells in the blood the condition is known as Sézary syndrome. Human papilloma virus has not been implicated in the pathogenesis of lymphoid malignancies. Adult T cell leukaemia/lymphoma is strongly associated with the retrovirus HTLV-1; this is rare in the UK but endemic in southern Japan. Coeliac disease may be complicated by the development of a high grade T cell tumour of the small intestine. Amyloidosis is a feature of some lymphomas but these are usually immunoblastic and of B cell type.

132. A. F
   B. F
   C. T
   D. T
   E. T

Raised intracranial pressure is associated with a number of systemic effects and these are largely the result of pressure effects on the hypothalamus and brain stem with autonomic overreactivity. This leads to systemic hypertension, bradycardia and pulmonary oedema. Supratentorial space-occupying lesions are associated with tentorial herniation and this in turn causes haemorrhage into the midbrain and pons. Papilloedema is a useful clinical sign of raised intracranial pressure.

133. A. F
   B. T
   C. T
   D. F
   E. T

Increased cerebrospinal fluid (CSF) volume may occur following cerebral infarction but this is *secondary* or compensatory hydrocephalus. The Arnold Chiari malformation is a congenital abnormality associated with spina bifida; blockage to CSF flow in this condition occurs at the level of the fourth ventricle. Colloid cysts of the third ventricle block the foramen of Monro and are associated with intermittent obstruction to CSF flow; this may be associated with hydrocephalus. Parkinson's disease is a degenerative disorder in which there is selective and progressive destruction of neurones in the substantia nigra; there is no abnormality of CSF flow. Aqueduct stenosis is a congenital abnormality which in some cases is an X-linked disorder; this condition is associated with impairment of CSF flow between the third and fourth ventricles.

134. A. F
  B. T
  C. T
  D. F
  E. F

Alzheimer's disease is the most common form of primary dementia. It is characterized histologically by the presence of senile plaques and neurofibrillary tangles. Progressive multifocal leucoencephalopathy is a demyelinating disorder caused by papova viruses in immunosuppressed individuals. Multiple sclerosis is the most common of the CNS demyelinating disorders. Huntington's disease is an autosomal dominant condition characterized by selective atrophy of the caudate nucleus. Hepatic encephalopathy is a metabolic disorder associated with liver failure; histological changes are minimal.

135. A. T
  B. T
  C. F
  D. F
  E. F

Acute diffuse proliferative glomerulonephritis most often follows pharyngitis that has resulted from group A haemolytic streptococci of types 12, 4 or 1. However, it is associated with a variety of other microorganisms, including viruses and malaria. Histologically the glomeruli are diffuse, enlarged and hypercellular with large numbers of neutrophils and macrophages. (Diffuse thickening of the basement membrane is seen in membranous glomerulonephritis.) Antiglomerular capillary basement membrane antibody is found in Goodpasture's sydrome. Acute diffuse proliferative glomerulonephritis in children is usually self-limiting with complete recovery and only a very small minority develop crescentic glomerulonephritis.

136. A. F
  B. T
  C. F
  D. T
  E. F

Infective endocarditis is associated with focal glomerulonephritis in approximately 20% of cases but this condition is *not* associated with pyelonephritis. Many structural and functional abnormalities in the urinary tract such as vesicoureteric reflux are associated with a predisposition to pyelonephritis. This is also the case for diabetes mellitus where there is a general susceptibility to infection. Gout causes tubulointerstitial injury but this is not usually associated with pyelonephritis. Amyloidosis usually affects the glomeruli and small blood vessels within the renal parenchyma; it is not associated with ascending infection.

137. A. F
  B. T
  C. T
  D. F
  E. T

Carcinomas arising in the bladder are most frequently of transitional cell type with a pseudostratified histological appearance. The bulk of such tumours are low grade, papillary neoplasms. Bladder tumours are seen with increased frequency in patients with *Schistosoma haematobium* infection, although in such individuals the tumour is usually a squamous cell carcinoma. There is an association with other environmental factors and an increased incidence is noted in workers in the rubber industry but there is no apparent increased risk in coal workers.

138. A. F
  B. F
  C. T
  D. F
  E. T

Testicular teratoma most frequently occurs in the 20–30-year age range. These are of germ cell origin but unlike ovarian teratomas they are rarely benign. They are not radiosensitive (cf. seminoma) and are usually treated by combination chemotherapy. Many teratomas with yolk sac differentiation express α-fetoprotein which can be used as a serum tumour marker.

139. A. T
  B. F
  C. T
  D. T
  E. F

Paget's disease of bone is characterized by increased bone turnover in which there is intense activity of osteoclasts and osteoblasts. It is generally associated with normal serum calcium and phosphate levels although alkaline phosphatase levels are elevated. Vitamin D deficiency causes osteomalacia and rickets and is not involved in the pathogenesis of Paget's disease. Osteosarcomas and other malignant tumours develop in a small proportion of patients with Paget's disease and high output cardiac failure is occasionally seen in individuals with extensive Paget's disease.

140. A. T
  B. F
  C. F
  D. T
  E. F

Ewing's sarcoma is a highly malignant tumour affecting the long bones of children and young adults. Its histogenesis remains uncertain but it is *not* derived from chondrocytes. (Tumours of chondroid tissue are referred to as either chondromas or chondrosarcomas.) Unlike neuroblastoma which also occurs in children, Ewing's sarcoma is not associated with raised urinary catecholamines. Many cases of Ewing's sarcoma show a reciprocal translocation between chromosomes 11 and 22. Ewing's sarcoma is treated by combination chemotherapy and surgery.

141. A. F
     B. T
     C. T
     D. F
     E. T

Rheumatoid arthritis is a common systemic inflammatory disease which predominantly affects the joints. It is characterized by inflammation and hyperplasia of the synovium and this is followed by destruction of articular surfaces. There is a female : male ratio of approximately 4 : 1. Circulating immune complexes (rheumatoid factors) can be identified in almost 90% of patients and these are thought to be important in the pathogenesis of the disease. Predisposition to rheumatoid arthritis is associated with HLA-DR4 (HLA-B27 is associated with seronegative arthritis, in particular ankylosing spondylitis). Felty's syndrome is a combination of rheumatoid arthritis and splenomegaly; this is associated with granulocytopenia and infection.

142. A. T
     B. F
     C. T
     D. T
     E. F

Cervical intraepithelial neoplasia (CIN) is a precursor for invasive squamous carcinoma of cervix. Human papilloma viruses have been implicated in its aetiology and there is a strong association between the development of CIN and level of sexual activity. The cellular abnormalities can be detected by cytology in cervical smear specimens and this forms the basis for the National Cytology Screening Programme. Females who were exposed *in utero* to diethylstilboestrol, a synthetic oestrogenic agent, are prone to developing vaginal adenosis but not CIN.

143. A. T
      B. F
      C. T
      D. F
      E. T

Paget's disease of the breast is infiltration of the nipple by malignant tumour adjacent to underlying *in situ* or invasive carcinoma; this may be the presenting feature of some breast cancers. Carcinomas most frequently occur in the upper outer quadrant of the breast. Over 60% of tumours express hormone receptors (oestrogen and progesterone receptors) and approximately 30% show clinical response to hormone therapy. The most common form of invasive carcinoma is infiltrating ductal carcinoma. Ductal carcinoma *in situ* has an excellent prognosis and can be treated by mastectomy alone.

144. A. F
      B. T
      C. T
      D. T
      E. F

Exophthalmos is seen in Graves' disease but not in Hashimoto's thyroiditis. Hashimoto's disease is an autoimmune condition in which the thyroid gland is infiltrated by chronic inflammatory cells and thyroid follicular cells become enlarged with a granular cytoplasm (Hürthle cell change). It is associated with the presence of circulating antimicrosomal and antithyroglobulin antibodies. B cell lymphomas arise in the thyroid in about 2% of patients with Hashimoto's thyroiditis. Iodine deficiency is responsible for endemic goitre in some parts of the world; this does not cause thyroiditis.

145. A. F
     B. F
     C. F
     D. T
     E. T

Papillary carcinoma of thyroid is usually seen in young adults. The tumours are derived from thyroid epithelium (C cell tumours are so-called medullary carcinomas). Papillary carcinomas are 'cold nodules' which do not show evidence of hyperfunction. Papillary carcinomas spread early to lymph nodes in the neck including those in the cervical chains and lymphadenopathy may be a presenting feature in some individuals. In common with other papillary tumours these neoplasms frequently show foci of dystrophic calcification in the form of calcispherites (psammoma bodies).

146. A. F
     B. T
     C. T
     D. F
     E. T

Primary hyperparathyroidism is most frequently caused by a functional parathyroid adenoma; carcinoma of the parathyroid accounts for less than 2% of all cases. It may occur as part of MEN-1 and MEN-2 syndromes. Excessive secretion of parathormone leads to increased bone turnover and development of bone disease where the marrow space becomes filled with fibrous tissue in which there is cystic degeneration (osteitis fibrosa cystica). The resultant hypercalcaemia is associated with metastatic calcification and the development of nephrocalcinosis and renal calculi. Hyperparathyroidism occurs in chronic renal failure but in this condition hypersecretion of parathormone occurs because the glands are stimulated by chronic hypocalcaemia; this is referred to as *secondary* hyperparathyroidism.

147. A. F
     B. T
     C. T
     D. F
     E. F

Dermatitis herpetiformis is characterized histologically by subepidermal bulla formation while in pemphigus vulgaris the bullae tend to be intraepidermal. Erythema nodosum is a vasculitic condition involving the dermis and subcutis. Lichen planus is associated with vacuolar degeneration to basal keratinocytes but this does not lead to bullous formation. Psoriasis is a hyperplastic disorder of the epidermis in which there is elongation of the rete ridges.

148. A. F
     B. F
     C. T
     D. F
     E. T

Squamous papillomas are benign lesions most commonly of viral origin (simple viral warts). Seborrhoeic keratosis is another form of benign squamous cell proliferation which is also referred to as basal cell papilloma. Keratoacanthomas are benign tumour-like lesions which can be mistaken clinically for squamous cell carcinomas; these are self-limiting and may also be of viral aetiology. Actinic keratosis and Bowen's disease both show varying degrees of keratinocyte dysplasia and carry a risk of development of invasive squamous cell carcinoma.

149. A. T
     B. F
     C. F
     D. T
     E. T

Molluscum contagiosum is caused by a pox virus. Verruca vulgaris (common viral wart) and condyloma accuminatum (genital wart) are both caused by subtypes of human papilloma virus. Impetigo is a superficial skin infection caused by *Staphylococcus aureus* or by haemolytic streptococci. Herpes gestationis is a bullous disorder that occurs during pregnancy and appears to have an autoimmune basis; it is not related to viral infection.

150. A. T
B. F
C. F
D. T
E. F

Specific proteins can be identified in tissue sections using immunohistochemistry. In tissue extracts they can be detected using Western blotting. Northern blotting is used to identify specific RNA transcripts and *in situ* hybridization is used to localize DNA or RNA in tissue sections. The polymerase chain reaction is used to enhance the amount of specific RNA or DNA fragment in tissue samples prior to their detection.

Clinical Biochemistry – Answers

151. A. T
B. T
C. F
D. F
E. T

Loss of water without sodium is unusual. Selective water depletion occurs when the loss of water exceeds that of sodium. Diabetic ketoacidosis causes an osmotic diuresis, leading to losses of both sodium and water. Administration of lithium salts can cause nephrogenic diabetes insipidus while vasopressin administration will cause water retention. Unconscious patients are unable, and dysphagic subjects may be unwilling, to respond adequately to thirst.

152. A. T
B. F
C. T
D. F
E. T

Sodium is the main cation of extracellular fluid while potassium is the main cation in intracellular fluid. Aldosterone stimulates sodium reabsorption in the distal tubule and aldosterone secretion rates increase postoperatively. Plasma sodium concentrations are a poor indicator of sodium balance, often being normal despite significant sodium depletion. Hyponatraemia can occur without deficits in body sodium if excess water is retained, e.g. because of inappropriate antidiuretic hormone secretion as a result of carcinoma of the bronchus. Cortisol has mineralocorticoid activity and thus sodium retention occurs in Cushing's syndrome.

153.   A.   F
   B.   F
   C.   F
   D.   T
   E.   F

Osmolality is a measure of solute particles per kg solvent while *osmolarity* is solute per litre. Low-molecular weight substances contribute more particles per unit mass than high-molecular weight substances; sodium and its associated anions contribute more than 90% of serum osmolality. Increased osmolality stimulates antidiuretic hormone (ADH) secretion. Osmolality is usually normal when hyponatraemia is caused by a decreased fractional water content of serum (hyperproteinaemia or hypertriglyceridaemia). In psychogenic polydipsia the osmolality is normal or reduced.

154.   A.   F
   B.   F
   C.   T
   D.   F
   E.   T

Addison's disease is primary adrenal failure; therefore adrenocorticotrophic hormone (ACTH) levels are high and these are associated with skin pigmentation. Lack of mineralocorticoids leads to salt and water loss and hyponatraemia and uraemia can occur but are not inevitable features unless severe disease is present. Hyperkalaemia and metabolic acidosis (not alkalosis) occur as a result of a failure of aldosterone-mediated distal tubular electrolyte exchange.

155.   A.   T
   B.   F
   C.   T
   D.   F
   E.   F

Insulin infusion increases cell uptake of potassium by increasing membrane Na^+/K^+-ATPase activity. Hyperkalaemia stimulates while hypokalaemia inhibits aldosterone secretion. Cardiac arrhythmias are important toxic effects of hyperkalaemia, high-peaked T waves being an early manifestation. Potassium depletion tends to produce alkalosis as H^+ ions are preferentially excreted in exchange for sodium by the distal tubule of the kidney. Loop diuretics, such as frusemide, increases losses, while aldosterone antagonists, such as amiloride, inhibit sodium reabsorption and potassium secretion in the distal tubule.

156. A. F
        B. T
        C. F
        D. F
        E. T

The renin–angiotensin system is the main controlling mechanism of aldosterone secretion, angiotensin II being the major stimulus. However, adrenocorticotrophic hormone (ACTH) produces transient increases in aldosterone secretion. Hyponatraemia stimulates renin and thus aldosterone secretion. Aldosterone increases as a result of changes in angiotensinogen II when subjects assume an upright posture. Hypovolaemia is a potent stimulus for renin secretion.

157. A. T
        B. T
        C. F
        D. F
        E. F

Blood pH is reduced in uncompensated metabolic acidosis, either because H^+ concentration is increased or because of loss of base. Plasma bicarbonate is reduced, either directly or because excess H^+ ions are buffered by bicarbonate. Excess H^+ ions stimulate the respiratory centre, lowering $P\text{co}_2$ and thus compensating for the acidosis by reducing the $P\text{co}_2$: bicarbonate ratio. Plasma potassium tends to be high in metabolic acidosis because of intracellular buffering and retention of K^+ in preference to H^+ by the distal renal tubules. The $P\text{o}_2$ is not reduced.

158. A. F
     B. F
     C. F
     D. T
     E. F

The anion gap is the difference between the concentration of principal cations (Na^+ and K^+) and anions (Cl^- and HCO_3^-) in plasma; in health this is 14–18 mmol/l. It is increased when an additional acidic anion, e.g. lactate, is present. Lactic acidosis is a recognized but rare complication of biguanide therapy. In MCAD deficiency excess dicarboxylic acids and medium-chain acyl-CoA esters are produced after prolonged fasting. Lactate is produced mainly in muscles and metabolized in the liver; it may thus accumulate in hepatic disease. In McArdle's disease (muscle phosphorylase deficiency) there is a failure to produce lactate on exercise.

159. A. F
     B. F
     C. F
     D. T
     E. T

Type I renal tubular acidosis (RTA) is usually inherited but may also be caused by autoimmune disorders, conditions which cause nephrocalcinosis, and by drugs and other renal diseases. Proximal tubular bicarbonate reabsorption is the primary abnormality in type II RTA while distal tubular H^+ secretion is defective in type I. This results in increased K^+ secretion, serum potassium usually being low, in contrast to other causes of metabolic acidosis. Chloride reabsorption is increased, the anion gap remaining normal. Hypercalciuria occurs, leading to calcium mobilization from bone.

160. A. T
      B. F
      C. T
      D. T
      E. F

Creatinine clearance is widely used as a clinical measure of glomerular filtration rate (GFR), since it is an endogenous substance and does not have to be injected. However, it overestimates values in end-stage renal disease, tubular secretion of creatinine occurring when serum concentrations are high. Both inulin and ethylenediamine tetra-acetic acid (EDTA) are excreted unchanged without tubular secretion or absorption. Radiolabelled EDTA is easier to estimate than inulin. Urea clearance has been used in the past although values are low because tubular reabsorption occurs, particularly when urinary flow rates are reduced. Para-aminohippuric acid excretion measures renal blood flow.

161. A. F
      B. F
      C. T
      D. T
      E. F

Urea, an end-product of amino acid metabolism, is synthesized in the liver. Plasma concentrations are partly determined by dietary protein intake and very low values are found normally in vegans. Digestion and absorption of proteins often produces mild uraemia following gastrointestinal bleeds. Mild uraemia is most commonly caused by congestive cardiac failure because of decreased renal perfusion. The glomerular filtration rate (GFR) may fall to approximately 30 ml/min without plasma urea concentrations increasing.

162. A. T
     B. T
     C. F
     D. F
     E. F

The liver is the main organ of gluconeogenesis although the kidney also contributes, particularly during prolonged starvation. Erythropoietin is a renal hormone which stimulates production of red blood cells. The kidney excretes water-soluble metabolic waste products while bilirubin, which is lipophilic, is conjugated in the liver and excreted in bile. The liver synthesizes 25-hydroxycholecalciferol which is further hydroxylated by the kidney to 1,25-dihydroxycholecalciferol, the active hormone derived from vitamin D. Angiotensinogen is secreted by the liver, the kidney producing renin.

163. A. T
     B. F
     C. F
     D. T
     E. T

Metabolic acidosis is common in chronic renal failure, mainly as a result of reduced excretion of H^+ and impaired renal bicarbonate regeneration. Compounds with a molecular weight of 1200–1500 Daltons ('middle molecules') are thought to cause toxaemia. Oliguria occurs in dehydration and acute renal failure while polyuria is common in chronic renal failure because the solute load per nephron is increased. Hyperprolactinaemia and reduced gonadal sex steroid production occur and impotence and oligomenorrhoea or amenorrhoea may result. Increased alkaline phosphatase activity is seen if renal osteodystrophy occurs.

164. A. T
      B. F
      C. T
      D. F
      E. F

Hypoalbuminaemia occurs because of heavy urinary protein loss. For this reason total T_4 levels are low although free T_4 is usually normal. The resulting reduced plasma oncotic pressure appears to stimulate hepatic synthesis of several proteins including albumin, apolipoprotein B and α_2-macroglobulin. Serum albumin does not rise as it is a small protein which is excreted by the abnormally permeable kidney, while larger proteins are usually retained. In nephrotic syndrome urinary protein excretion typically exceeds $3.5\,g/m^2$ body surface area.

165. A. F
      B. F
      C. T
      D. F
      E. F

Most patients with a single calcium-containing stone eventually form another, the average rate being one every 2–3 years. Calcium phosphate precipitation is favoured by alkaline urine while urate precipitation is favoured by acid urine. Oxalate stones occur in patients with fat malabsorption because unabsorbed fat binds Ca^{2+} in the gut lumen, leading to increased oxalate solubility and absorption. Urate stones are radiotranslucent. Cystinuria is a transport disorder of cystine, ornithine, arginine and lysine.

166. A. T
      B. T
      C. F
      D. T
      E. T

Approximately half circulating calcium is ionized, 45% protein bound, mainly to albumin, and 3% complexed with citrate. Alkalosis increases protein binding of Ca^{2+} while acidosis has the opposite effect. Ca^{2+} has many metabolic actions including effects on neuromuscular excitability, cell membrane structure and transport, intracellular enzyme activity and, as a second messenger, hormone action.

167. A. T
     B. T
     C. F
     D. T
     E. T

PTH is secreted in response to falls in serum Ca^{2+} concentration. The interaction of PTH with membrane receptors initiates a series of intracellular events which mediate hormone actions. These include increased distal tubular reabsorption of calcium, decreased phosphate reabsorption and reduced bicarbonate reabsorption. Thus, hypophosphataemia and metabolic acidosis may occur in primary hyperparathyroidism.

168. A. T
     B. F
     C. T
     D. T
     E. T

Reduced synthesis of 1,25-dihydroxycholecalciferol and phosphate retention are important in the pathogenesis of hypocalcaemia in end-stage renal disease. Reduced bone mass occurs in osteoporosis without changes in serum calcium. Parathyroid hormone (PTH) releases calcium from bone, while magnesium is required for PTH secretion and action. Several factors may contribute to hypocalcaemia in pancreatitis, including protein exudation into the peritoneal cavity, Ca^{2+} sequestration by fatty acids released from omental fat as a result of lipase activity, and hormonal disturbances such as calcitonin release.

169. A. F
B. T
C. T
D. F
E. T

Secondary hyperparathyroidism is caused by reduced 1,25-dihydroxycholecalciferol formation and results in increased parathyroid hormone (PTH) secretion and parathyroid hyperplasia. Hypercalcaemia does not occur unless autonomous secretion occurs in a gland. Malignant tumours produce hypercalcaemia by several mechanisms including bone lysis, production of PTH-like substances and prostaglandin secretion. Sarcoidosis causes hypercalcaemia because of increased 1-hydroxylation of vitamin D in granulomas. Osteomalacia is characterized by defective mineralization of bone as a result of vitamin D deficiency and serum calcium levels tend to be low. Thiazide diuretics reduce renal calcium excretion.

170. A. F
B. T
C. T
D. F
E. F

Vitamin D intoxication causes increased serum phosphate levels by facilitating phosphate absorption in the intestine. Increased cellular uptake of serum phosphate by depleted tissues occurs in patients given parenteral nutrition and supplements may be necessary. Patients with diabetic ketoacidosis often have high levels at presentation but these fall during treatment as a result of increased tissue uptake. Hypercalcaemia may be seen in Paget's disease if patients are immobilized but phosphate levels are normal. Growth hormone increases renal tubular phosphate reabsorption, increasing serum phosphate.

171. A. F
B. T
C. T
D. F
E. F

Magnesium ions are essential for normal myocardial function and magnesium depletion is associated with atherogenesis. However, myocardial infarction does not cause magnesium depletion. Parathyroid hormone (PTH) increases renal tubular magnesium reabsorption. Magnesium deficiency occurs in various states associated with poor nutrition, including alcoholism. Retention of magnesium may complicate chronic renal failure. Increased release of cellular magnesium occurs in diabetic ketoacidosis and serum levels are usually raised.

172. A. F
B. F
C. T
D. T
E. T

Very low density lipoproteins (VLDL) are assembled in the liver. ApoAI occurs in high density lipoprotein (HDL) while apoB is the major protein of low density lipoprotein (LDL). Low density lipoprotein contains the majority of circulating cholesterol. Chylomicrons transport dietary fat from the intestine, the triglyceride content being cleared by lipoprotein lipase in adipose tissue, muscle and the lactating mammary gland. Chylomicrons and VLDL contain apoB when secreted and acquire apoE and apoC-II, which are necessary for metabolism of these lipoproteins, from HDL in the circulation.

173. A. F
       B. F
       C. T
       D. T
       E. T

Familial hypercholesterolaemia (FH) is an autosomal dominant condition, homozygotes being more severely affected than heterozygotes. Tendon xanthomas occur in FH while eruptive xanthomas are found in severe hypertriglyceridaemia. ApoE is important in the metabolism of VLDL to LDL. The common phenotype is E3/E3, E2/E2 being commonly found in type III hyperlipoproteinaemia. Elevated LDL cholesterol is an important modifiable risk factor for coronary heart disease, LDL being found in arterial fatty streaks, which lead to atherosclerotic lesions. Type I hyperlipidaemia is a result of severely impaired catabolic clearance of chylomicrons and is either caused by a deficiency of the clearing enzyme, lipoprotein lipase, or the apoprotein which activates the enzyme, apoC- II.

174. A. T
       B. T
       C. F
       D. F
       E. T

Beta-blocking drugs increase VLDL levels, particularly in patients with pre-existing hypertriglyceridaemia, and decrease HDL cholesterol concentrations. Ethanol can cause increased lipolysis in adipose tissue, so releasing non-esterified fatty acids (NEFA) to the blood and hence the liver. Ethanol, rather than fatty acids, is oxidized by hepatocytes and triglyceride synthesis is increased. Hypothyroidism and diabetes mellitus (not diabetes insipidus) are causes of secondary hyperlipidaemia. Cholestasis leads to hypercholesterolaemia by interfering with the excretion of biliary sterols.

175. A. F
B. T
C. T
D. T
E. F

The resting metabolic rate rises as body weight increases. Basal insulin levels and responses to test meals are increased in obesity; impaired glucose tolerance and non-insulin-dependent diabetes mellitus are more prevalent. A 10% increase in body fat is associated with a 6 mm rise in diastolic blood pressure. The incidence of osteoarthritis is increased, particularly in weight-bearing joints.

176. A. F
B. T
C. F
D. F
E. T

Insulin regulates intracellular events after binding with receptors on cell membranes. It promotes lipogenesis and inhibits lipolysis. Ketone bodies are derived from NEFA, plasma levels of which are lowered by insulin which also inhibits the ketogenic effect of glucagon. Alanine is released from muscle in insulin deficiency and transported to the liver where it is a gluconeogenic substrate. Insulin inhibits the glycogenolytic effect of glucagon.

177. A. F
B. T
C. F
D. F
E. T

Type 1 (insulin-dependent) diabetes mellitus (IDDM) is due to destruction of B (β) cells; A (α) cells produce glucagon. IDDM is associated with the HLA antigens DR3 and DR4. Approximately 70% of patients have circulating islet cell antibodies at presentation although these decrease with time. IDDM typically presents in patients less than 30 years old with peak incidences in childhood. Ketosis is common at presentation.

178. A. F
  B. F
  C. T
  D. T
  E. F

Type 2 diabetes mellitus (NIDDM) generally presents over the age of 40 years although it can occur in young adults (maturity-onset diabetes mellitus of the young; MODY). Many but not all patients are obese. Inheritance is a more important factor in the development of type 2 than type 1 diabetes. In obese NIDDM patients insulin secretion is greater than in non-obese non-diabetic subjects but less than in non-diabetic obese subjects. Insulin is sometimes needed to control NIDDM patients.

179. A. T
  B. F
  C. F
  D. T
  E. T

Leucocytosis is inevitable in diabetic ketoacidosis (DKA), correlating with blood ketone levels and is not necessarily caused by an infection. Hyponatraemia is common because of osmotic shifts of water from cells to extracellular fluid, diluting sodium. Increased secretion of counterregulatory hormones is a result of either a precipitating infection or the metabolic disturbance. Kussmaul breathing results from stimulation of the respiratory centre by the acidosis. Hypovolaemia is caused by an osmotic diuresis which occurs because the renal threshold for glucose reabsorption is exceeded.

180. A. T
   B. F
   C. T
   D. F
   E. F

More than half of patients with HONK are undiagnosed diabetic patients. The mortality is over 50%. Severe dehydration is common and hypernatraemia occurs in most patients. Minor degrees of ketosis without acidosis are common. Insulin is needed to correct the metabolic state.

181. A. F
   B. T
   C. T
   D. T
   E. F

Impaired glucose tolerance is a recognized side-effect of thiazides. Large tumours may cause hypoglycaemia, either because of increased glucose uptake or because they produce substances such as growth factors which have insulin-like actions. Cortisol, an important counterregulatory hormone, is deficient in Addison's disease. Alcohol inhibits gluconeogenesis and increases insulin release in response to an oral glucose load. Nicotinic acid inhibits lipolysis but rebound increases in non-esterified fatty acid (NEFA) levels follow and may worsen control in diabetes by NEFA being preferentially oxidized, decreasing glucose utilization.

182. A. T
   B. F
   C. T
   D. T
   E. T

Proinsulin is converted into insulin and C-peptide and thus equimolar amounts of each are secreted. There are greater species differences in C-peptide than in insulin. Insulin production is defective in type 1 diabetes and therefore C-peptide levels are low, unlike type 2 diabetes. Sulphonylureas enhance the release of insulin, and thus C-peptide, from the pancreas. Insulinoma patients have C-peptide levels which parallel those of insulin while patients with factitious hypoglycaemia caused by exogenous insulin administration suppress endogenous insulin and thus C-peptide.

183. A. F
     B. F
     C. T
     D. T
     E. F

Type I (von Gierke) glycogen storage disease is caused by glucose-6-phosphatase deficiency while debrancher enzyme is defective in type III (Cori) disease. The liver, intestine and kidney are affected. Hypoglycaemia, hepatomegaly and lactic acidosis are recognized features of the disease.

184. A. F
     B. T
     C. T
     D. T
     E. T

Three enzyme deficiencies, galactose-1-phosphate uridyl transferase, galactokinase and uridine diphosphate galactose-4-epimerase, cause galactosaemia, clinical manifestations being most severe with galactose-1-phosphate uridyl transferase deficiency. Cataract formation is caused by a metabolite, galactitol, accumulating in the lens and attracting water osmotically. Galactose accumulation in renal tubules can cause Fanconi syndrome, interfering with amino acid reabsorption. Galactose, a reducing substance, is excreted. Severe liver damage occurs although the mechanism is unclear.

185. A. F
     B. F
     C. F
     D. F
     E. T

Starch is the most abundant carbohydrate in the diet, small amounts of lactose and sucrose also being ingested. Amylase hydrolyses $\alpha(1\rightarrow4)$ linkages in starch not $\alpha(1\rightarrow6)$ linkages, which are chain branch points. Lactose is a disaccharide of glucose and galactose, sucrose is a disaccharide of glucose and fructose. Fructose is passively absorbed by a mediated mechanism. Bacterial fermentation of non-absorbed carbohydrates produces several products including hydrogen which, after absorption, is excreted by the lungs.

186. A. F
     B. T
     C. T
     D. F
     E. T

Absorption of small peptides accounts for some amino acid absorption. Similar specific amino acid transport processes occur in the small intestine and renal tubule. The body can convert phenylalanine to tyrosine but not vice versa. Trypsin, the main proteolytic enzyme of the pancreas is most active at an alkaline pH. Increased urinary nitrogen excretion after operation is part of a general catabolic response to injury.

187. A. T
     B. T
     C. F
     D. F
     E. T

Vitamin E is thought to prevent fatty acid and possibly cholesterol peroxidation. Vitamin A is necessary for the normal differentiation of epithelia. Riboflavin is a coenzyme for oxidation–reduction reactions, being incorporated into flavin adenine dinucleotide. Pyridoxine is a coenzyme for decarboxylation and transamination reactions while nicotinic acid is a component of NAD and NADP. Folic acid is a coenzyme in methylation reactions leading to thymine synthesis.

188. A. T
       B. T
       C. T
       D. T
       E. T

Hyperglycaemia results from impaired glucose tolerance and because there is less hepatic glycogen synthesis. In the liver excess glucose may be converted to fat which may accumulate. Lipaemia occurs if the infusion rate of lipid exceeds the clearance rate. Hyponatraemia is common, the causes being multifactorial, e.g. prior losses of sodium and water retention. Hyperchloraemic metabolic acidosis may result from the administration of amino acids in the form of hydrochlorides.

189. A. T
       B. F
       C. F
       D. F
       E. F

Impaired hydroxylation of phenylalanine may result from several enzyme defects, classic phenylketonuria resulting from deficient phenylalanine hydroxylase deficiency. The enzyme normally is present mainly in the liver although the kidney also shows activity. The gene locus for the apoenzyme has been mapped to chromosome 12. Tyrosine is the product of normal enzymatic hydroxylation of phenylalanine and levels are either normal or reduced. The objective of therapy is to maintain normal blood levels: low levels have been associated with poor growth and neurological symptoms.

190. A. F
B. T
C. F
D. F
E. T

Ammonium chloride loading is a test of urinary acidification and is abnormal in type I renal tubular acidosis. Triglyceride tolerance and other assessments of fat absorption such as faecal fat excretion or $^{14}CO_2$ excretion after a labelled fat meal may be abnormal when pancreatic lipases are deficient or if mucosal disease is present. D-Xylose absorption is an investigation for jejunal mucosal abnormalities and breath hydrogen analysis reflects bacterial carbohydrate breakdown in the gut. The ^{14}C-PABA (para-aminobenzoic acid) excretion test depends on chymotrypsin which hydrolyses a synthetic substrate to release PABA, which is excreted in urine.

191. A. F
B. T
C. T
D. T
E. F

Intestinal lactase activity is highest in early infancy, falling with weaning. Levels are low in most ethnic groups in adult life although activity is retained by the majority of Caucasians. Undigested lactose is broken down by colonic bacteria to short-chain fatty acids and various gases including hydrogen, often causing diarrhoea with acidic stools in children. Secondary hypolactasia may occur in several enteropathies, including gastroenteritis and coeliac disease. Increased breath hydrogen excretion following a lactose load is usual in hypolactasia although some subjects appear to lack hydrogen-producing colonic microorganisms.

192. A. F
 B. F
 C. F
 D. T
 E. F

Amylase activities >10 times the upper limit of normal are virtually diagnostic of acute pancreatitis while values >5 times the upper limit may occur in diabetic ketoacidosis, perforated peptic ulcer and other acute abdominal disorders. Urinary amylase is increased, sometimes after the serum amylase returns to normal. Diabetes mellitus occasionally complicates acute haemorrhagic pancreatitis. Methaemalbuminaemia develops in some cases of acute pancreatitis, presumably as a result of proteolytic breakdown of haemoglobin. Pancreatitis may occur as a complication of severe hypertriglyceridaemia, not hypercholesterolaemia. The reason hypertriglyceridaemia causes pancreatitis is not clear but is possibly due to the interference of large lipoprotein particles with the pancreatic microcirculation.

193. A. F
 B. T
 C. F
 D. T
 E. F

Paraproteins are produced by single clones of B cells and the molecules are identical. Approximately 20% of cases of myeloma tumours produce only light chains which are small enough to be excreted in urine as Bence–Jones protein. Such paraproteins may not be detected in serum. Benign paraproteins occur although the diagnosis can only be made after rigorous investigations to exclude malignant causes. Paraprotein bands are usually detected in the γ region on electrophoresis although a different migration may occur, particularly if the protein is immunoglobulin (Ig) A.

194. A. T
B. T
C. F
D. T
E. T

The concentrations of several serum proteins including α_1-antitrypsin increase in acute inflammation. It is the main protease inhibitor in serum. Many alleles of the gene have been recognized, MM being associated with normal serum concentrations and ZZ being most often associated with deficiency. Emphysema is thought to occur in deficiency states because elastase is not inhibited in the lung. Neonatal hepatitis is also a feature of deficiency and this may progress to cirrhosis.

195. A. F
B. T
C. T
D. F
E. T

Albumin is synthesized in the liver and hypoalbuminaemia is a feature of chronic hepatic diseases such as portal cirrhosis. Albumin transports several substances including unconjugated bilirubin, non-esterified fatty acids (NEFA), calcium and thyroxine. Prolonged venous stasis causes haemoconcentration. Albumin is the major determinant of plasma oncotic pressure and peripheral oedema may occur in analbuminaemia although it is not inevitable and is usually episodic. Reduced plasma volume occurs in hypoalbuminaemia, leading to increased renin and thus aldosterone secretion.

196. A. F
        B. F
        C. T
        D. T
        E. F

Hepatocytes synthesize many plasma proteins but immunoglobulins are produced by plasma cells. Primary bile acids are synthesized in the liver; secondary bile acids are formed from these by gut bacteria and then absorbed. The liver is the major site of gluconeogenesis and in starvation or diabetic ketoacidosis it produces ketone bodies from non-esterified fatty acids (NEFA), these being used as an alternative energy substrate to glucose, particularly by brain.
Urobilinogen is produced in the gut by bacteria from bilirubin and some is absorbed.

197. A. F
        B. T
        C. T
        D. F
        E. T

Most serum bilirubin in healthy subjects is unconjugated, conjugated bilirubin being excreted rapidly into bile. Phenobarbitone and phenytoin induce increased activity of conjugating enzymes. Haemolytic jaundice is caused by excessive erythrocyte breakdown and the resulting excess bilirubin in serum is unconjugated. Gilbert's disease is caused by defective hepatic uptake and conjugation of bilirubin. Dubin–Johnson syndrome is a rare defect of bilirubin excretion.

198. A. F
     B. T
     C. T
     D. F
     E. F

Creatine kinase occurs in brain and skeletal and cardiac muscle; hydroxybutyrate dehydrogenase is the cardiac isoenzyme of lactate dehydrogenase. Alkaline phosphatase is found in biliary epithelium and hepatocytes but is raised in serum in obstructive rather than in hepatocellular disease. Several tissues contain large amounts of aspartate aminotransferase and therefore increased serum activities are not specific for hepatocellular damage. Although alanine aminotransferase occurs in several tissues, increases in serum are more hepatospecific. '

199. A. T
     B. F
     C. T
     D. T
     E. F

In cholestasis, conjugation of bilirubin occurs but excretion is defective. Less bilirubin reaches the gut and less urobilinogen is formed. However, bilirubinuria may occur. Biliary enzymes, including γ-glutamyl transpeptidase, increase in serum, either because of increased synthesis or release from cell membranes. Osteomalacia is caused by reduced vitamin D absorption as a result of fat malabsorption and interruption to the enterohepatic circulation of bile salts. In addition, jaundice may reduce cutaneous synthesis of vitamin D. Increased blood ammonia levels occur in hepatocellular failure.

200. A. T
B. T
C. T
D. F
E. F

Wilson's disease is an inherited defect in the excretion of copper from hepatocytes into bile, usually accompanied by a decrease in hepatic caeruloplasmin synthesis. Copper accumulates in tissues including the kidney, causing aminoaciduria. Serum copper concentrations are usually lower than normal, the reduction in the copper transport protein caeruloplasmin somewhat offset by an increase in copper bound to albumin or amino acids. Diabetes mellitus can occur as a complication of haemochromatosis but not Wilson's disease.

201. A. T
B. F
C. T
D. F
E. T

Cholinesterase is synthesized in the liver and serum activity is often low in chronic diseases such as decompensated cirrhosis. It is not reduced by anaesthesia but the enzyme hydrolyses suxamethonium (scoline). Patients with congenital deficiency of cholinesterase suffer prolonged apnoea when scoline is administered during anaesthesia. Levels of cholinesterase are not affected by renal disease, but are reduced by poisoning with insecticides which contain organophosphates.

202. A. F
B. T
C. T
D. F
E. F

The prostatic isoenzyme of acid phosphatase is markedly inhibited by tartrate while the erythrocyte form is only slightly inhibited. Tartrate-labile acid phosphatase, unlike prostate specific antigen, is not elevated in benign prostatic hypertrophy but increases occur after rectal examination and in 90% of patients with skeletal metastases from prostatic carcinoma. Although total acid phosphatase may be increased in carcinoma of the breast and in Gaucher's disease this increase does not affect the tartrate-labile fraction.

203. A. F
B. F
C. F
D. T
E. F

Increased CK may result from causes other than myocardial infarction, such as intramuscular injections given to treat chest pain. Increases in CK-MB occur slightly earlier than total CK, the latter peaking at 24 hours post infarction. Continuing increases in CK in the absence of injections and skeletal muscle damage suggest infarct extension. Aspartate aminotransferase (AST) activity returns to normal after 72 hours while hydroxybutyrate dehydrogenase may be elevated after 6 days.

204. A. T
B. F
C. F
D. T
E. T

In resting adults growth hormone is often undetectable in serum between secretory bursts which last 1–2 hours. Secretion is stimulated by stress, hypoglycaemia, exercise and interleukin-1. Its secretion is controlled by a balance between the effects of two regulatory hypothalamic hormones: growth hormone releasing hormone and growth hormone release inhibiting hormone (somatostatin).

205.   A.   T
  B.   F
  C.   T
  D.   T
  E.   T

Acromegaly causes overgrowth of soft tissues and bones and
gigantism may result if it occurs before the epiphyses fuse.
Some tumours are composed of acidophil or chromophobe
cells. Sporadic cases of diabetes insipidus occur, as a result of
the local effects of the space-occupying lesion, while growth
hormone has anti-insulin effects. Galactorrhoea can occur
because hyperprolactinaemia is found in approximately 50%
of patients, either because of a mixed tumour or as a result of
interference by the tumour with dopamine-induced inhibition
of prolactin secretion.

206.   A.   F
  B.   F
  C.   F
  D.   T
  E.   F

There is a peak in serum luteinizing hormone (LH) prior to
ovulation. Interstitial cell-stimulating hormone is required for
Leydig cell function while follicle-stimulating hormone (FSH)
promotes seminiferous tubule development. Gonadotrophin
levels are raised in primary gonadal failure because of a lack
of negative feedback by gonadal hormones. Similarly,
gonadotrophins increase after the menopause. Clomiphene
induces secretion of gonadotrophin-releasing hormone and
thus gonadotrophins.

207.   A.   T
         B.   T
         C.   T
         D.   T
         E.   F

Osmolality is the main controlling mechanism for ADH
secretion although reduced plasma volume is a stimulant, even
if osmolality is reduced. Ectopic ADH release can occur, most
often as a result of a small cell bronchial carcinoma. Ethanol
is an inhibitor of ADH release. Chlorpropamide increases renal
sensitivity to ADH. Vasopressin increases the permeability of
the distal tubule and collecting duct enabling water to be
absorbed passively down the concentration gradient which is
present normally in the kidney.

208.   A.   T
         B.   T
         C.   F
         D.   T
         E.   F

Prolactin levels are raised by stress, including venepuncture.
To avoid this effect samples are best taken via a cannula,
allowing time for the stress of cannulation to pass. Drugs that
interfere with the inhibitory effect of dopamine, such as
chlorpromazine, cause hyperprolactinaemia. Elevated
prolactin levels inhibit ovulation. Lesions in the hypothalamus
or pituitary stalk may prevent hypothalamic dopamine
reaching the pituitary and inhibiting prolactin secretion.
Hyperprolactinaemia may occur in hypothyroidism, possibly
because of an effect of elevated thyrotrophin-releasing
hormone (TRH).

209. A. T
B. F
C. T
D. F
E. F

Dwarfism is a feature of cretinism, congenital hypothyroidism.
Receptors for free thyroid hormones are found in cell nuclei.
Some consider the effect on sex hormone binding globulin
(SHBG) levels to be a useful peripheral test of thyroid
function. Thyroid-stimulating hormone (RSH) levels may not
be elevated if hypothyroidism is secondary to pituitary
hypofunction. Graves' disease is thought to result from the
action of thyroid-stimulating antibodies which mimic the effect
of TSH.

210. A. F
B. F
C. T
D. F
E. F

Increased total thyroxine (T_4) occurs in pregnancy as a result
of increased synthesis of thyroxine-binding globulin (TBG);
however, free T_4 is not affected by changes in TBG and levels
tend to fall in the second and third trimesters because of
haemodilution resulting from water retention. Androgens
decrease TBG but have no effect on free T_4. Amiodarone is
an antiarrhthymic drug which decreases peripheral conversion
of T_4 to triiodothyronine (T_3), increasing T_4 levels. Rarely T_4
levels may be normal in thyrotoxicosis, high concentrations of
T_3 being found. Severe non-thyroidal illness often reduces T_4.

211.   A.   T
           B.   F
           C.   F
           D.   T
           E.   F

Glucocorticoids enhance gluconeogenesis and antagonize the peripheral effects of insulin. Increased levels may lead to diabetes mellitus. Glucocorticoids antagonize the action of antidiuretic hormone (ADH) on renal tubules. They increase neutrophils, lower lymphocyte and eosinophil counts and are anti-inflammatory. Glucocorticoids enhance angiotensinogen production and sensitize arterioles to the action of noradrenaline.

212.   A.   F
           B.   T
           C.   F
           D.   T
           E.   T

Cushing's syndrome is most commonly caused by adrenal hyperplasia resulting from increased pituitary adrenocorticotrophic hormone (ACTH) secretion. Oligomenorrhoea and impotence are symptoms. In the high dose dexamethasone test 90% of patients with pituitary-dependent disease show suppression of cortisol levels while adrenal adenomata do not suppress. Patients with simple obesity retain the circadian pattern of cortisol secretion, a normal response to hypoglycaemia and corticosteroid suppression by low dose dexamethasone. Hypokalaemia is more commonly a result of ectopic ACTH production than other causes of Cushing's syndrome.

213. A. F
B. F
C. T
D. T
E. T

Over 90% of cases of congenital adrenal hyperplasia are the result of 21-hydroxylase deficiency and salt loss occurs in 66% of these. Hypertension occurs in 11β-hydroxylase deficiency as a result of increased deoxycorticosterone synthesis. Hypokalaemia occurs in 17α-hydroxylase deficiency. The clinical presentation of cases is extremely variable, including sudden infant death, salt-losing crises, ambiguous genitalia, pseudoprecocious puberty, hirsutism, testicular tumour and infertility.

214. A. T
B. T
C. F
D. T
E. T

Most abnormalities of sex chromosomes cause primary amenorrhoea although secondary amenorrhoea may occur with a triple X chromosome. Prolactin interferes with gonadotroph release and probably also inhibits the action of gonadotrophins on the ovaries. Primary amenorrhoea is a feature of Kallman's syndrome (hypogonadotrophic hypogonadism). Appropriate pulsatile gonadotroph release from the pituitary is dependent on body weight. Sheehan's syndrome is secondary to postpartum infarction of the anterior pituitary.

215. A. T
   B. T
   C. F
   D. F
   E. T

The placenta produces a heat-stable alkaline phosphatase isoenzyme, the measurement of which has been used as a placental function test. Plasma urea decreases because plasma volume expands and glomerular filtration rate (GFR) increases. Serum cholesterol increases in pregnancy, all lipoprotein fractions being affected. Serum cortisol increases because the binding protein, transcortin, increases. Glycosuria in pregnancy may reflect a reduced renal threshold or gestational diabetes mellitus.

216. A. T
   B. T
   C. F
   D. T
   E. T

In phaeochromocytoma excess catecholamine secretion causes peripheral vasoconstriction. Increased serum calcium levels appear to have a direct vasoconstrictive effect. In Conn's syndrome (primary hyperaldosteronism) hypertension appears to be related to sodium retention. Hypertension, obesity and dyslipidaemia are commonly associated in NIDDM, probably all related to hyperinsulinaemia (Reaven's syndrome or syndrome X). There is no evidence for an increased incidence of hypertension in hypothyroidism.

217. A. T
   B. F
   C. F
   D. T
   E. F

Serum γ-glutamyl transpeptidase is a relatively sensitive indicator of excessive alcohol intake. In common with other agents which increase hepatic microsomal enzyme activities, alcohol increases serum high density lipoprotein (HDL)-cholesterol levels. Alcohol increases insulin release in response to an oral glucose load and may cause reactive hypoglycaemia; in addition, alcohol inhibits gluconeogenesis and may cause fasting hypoglycaemia. The mechanism of hypercortisolism in alcoholics is not clear. Hydrogen ion secretion by the stomach is induced by alcohol.

218. A. T
B. T
C. F
D. F
E. T

Lead interferes with several steps of porphyrin synthesis, and increased urinary excretion of δ-aminolaevulinic and coproporphyrin are characteristic. Neuropathic features of lead poisoning include encephalopathy in children and peripheral neuropathy in adults. Abdominal colic and pain also occur, without leucocytosis. Mild anaemia with basophilic stippling of erythrocytes is common. Aminoaciduria is a feature of poisoning with various heavy metals.

219. A. T
B. T
C. F
D. T
E. F

Vertigo, tinnitus and impairment of hearing are early symptoms of chronic salicylate intoxication. Acute overdose causes metabolic acidosis, partly due to retention of inorganic acids as a result of impaired renal function and partly due to impaired carbohydrate metabolism, resulting in accumulation of organic acids. Impaired renal function occurs because of dehydration and hypotension. There is no specific antidote but the renal clearance of salicylate is increased if the urine is alkalinized.

220. A. T
    B. F
    C. T
    D. T
    E. F

Paracetamol poisoning causes centrilobular hepatic necrosis, the toxic metabolite being *N*-acetyl *p*-benzoquinonimine, which can also cause renal damage. Small quantities of this metabolite are produced normally and it is detoxified by glutathione. However, this detoxification is saturated by acute overdoses. Hypoglycaemia occurs in hepatic failure as a result of reduced gluconeogenesis. Blood levels are best determined between 4 and 12 hours after ingestion.

221. A. F
    B. T
    C. F
    D. T
    E. T

Homovanillic acid is a metabolite of dopamine and excretion may be increased in neuroblastoma and malignant phaeochromocytoma. Carcinoid syndrome is a tumour of argentaffin cells which produce 5-hydroxytryptamine (serotonin) from which 5-hydroxyindole acetic acid is derived by oxidation. Plasma and platelet levels of serotonin are usually elevated. Carcinoid tumours also produce amines and multiple peptide hormones which are thought to mediate many of the pathological changes that are seen. Manifestations include cutaneous flushing, diarrhoea, valvular heart disease and, uncommonly, paroxysmal hypotension.

222. A. T
       B. T
       C. T
       D. F
       E. F

Impaired renal function occurs in pre-eclampsia and serum urate increases, roughly in proportion to the severity of the disease. Lesch–Nyhan syndrome is a rare inherited condition in which reconversion of purines to nucleotides is impaired and the formation of urate is thus increased. Hyperuricaemia is caused by increased cell turnover in myeloproliferative disorders. Colchicine inhibits the inflammatory response in gout but does not reduce serum urate levels. Renal tubular reabsorption of urate is reduced in the Fanconi syndrome.

223. A. F
       B. T
       C. F
       D. T
       E. T

Increased faecal protoporphyrin is a feature of variagate porphyria. Acute intermittent porphyria is caused by a partial defect in porphobilinogen deaminase which converts porphobilinogen to uroporphyrinogen. Increased production of δ-aminolaevulinic acid and porphobilinogen results, particularly during acute attacks. Aminolaevulinic acid causes neuropathic features. Cutaneous photosensitivity is not induced by excess porphobilinogen but occurs when increased porphyrins are present in skin. Oestrogens, in common with many other drugs, induce increased δ-aminolaevulinic acid synthetase activity, increasing the synthesis of toxic metabolites.

224. A. F
   B. F
   C. F
   D. T
   E. F

For data with a Gaussian distribution the range included by the mean ± 2 standard deviations includes 95% of the population. Sensitivity measures the incidence of positive results in patients known to have a disease and specificity measures the incidence of negative results in patients free of a disease. Efficiency is the number of positive and negative results as a percentage of the total. Precision measures reproducibility while accuracy is a measure of how close a result is to the true value.

225. A. F
   B. F
   C. F
   D. T
   E. F

By convention, reference ranges include 95% of values from a healthy population if the data have a Gaussian (normal) distribution. However some analytes, e.g. cholesterol, have a skewed distribution. Ranges may differ according to the method of analysis, gender and age. Repeated test results in healthy individuals sometimes show an occasional value outside the reference range while the majority fall within.

Haematology –
Answers

226. A. T
B. T
C. F
D. F
E. T

Iron deficiency and thalassaemias (both alpha and beta) are
microcytic. Anaemias of chronic disorder may be microcytic
or normocytic. Patients with thalassaemia traits may also be
iron deficient. The low serum iron of anaemia of chronic
disorder may mimic iron deficiency but the serum ferritin is
usually raised in this disorder. Sickle cell trait is not microcytic
unless the patient is, for example, also iron deficient. Renal
failure is usually associated with normochromic, normocytic
anaemia.

227. A. F
B. F
C. F
D. T
E. T

The normal newborn has a high haemoglobin (Hb) and is
macrocytic compared with normal children and adults. Most
of its Hb is fetal, but some adult Hb is often detectable at birth.
The Kleihauer test detects fetal Hb-containing red cells in the
maternal circulation, so will always be positive in the infant.
Circulating nucleated red cells, always abnormal in older
individuals, are often detectable in the blood of normal
neonates. (MCV is the abbreviation for mean cell volume.)

228. A. F
   B. F
   C. T
   D. T
   E. T

For Rh haemolytic disease of the newborn (HDN) to occur the mother must be Rh D negative and her fetus Rh D positive. Intrauterine transfusion can result in a full-term, healthy infant, but exchange transfusion after birth is used to treat established HDN. Phototherapy with blue light accelerates bilirubin breakdown and slows down the rate of rise of bilirubin in affected infants. Any inherited haemolytic anaemia may cause HDN. Rhesus negativity is rare in the Far East while glucose-6-phosphate dehydrogenase (G6PD) deficiency, an inherited haemolytic anaemia, is common.

229. A. T
   B. T
   C. F
   D. F
   E. F

Postpartum injection of anti-D in Rh D negative mothers with Rh D positive infants reduces the risk of sensitization by a transplacental bleed. First babies are rarely affected. The smaller the family size, the smaller the number of affected babies, and families are significantly smaller now than 20 years ago.

230. A. T
   B. F
   C. F
   D. F
   E. T

Both folic acid and B_{12} deficiency cause macrocytic anaemia. Bone marrow examination reveals the megaloblastic changes in red and white cell precursors. B_{12} deficiency may cause severe neuropathy and subacute combined degeneration of the cord. Coeliac disease may result in malabsorption of both folate and iron; macrocytosis may then not be obvious and the *mean* cell volume (MCV) may be normal. Even vegetarians may suffer malabsorption severe enough to result in folate deficiency, but this would indeed be bad luck!

231. A. F
B. T
C. F
D. F
E. T

Pernicious anaemia (PA) is an autoimmune disease which results in failure of gastric cells to secrete enough intrinsic factor, without which B_{12} cannot be absorbed in the terminal ileum. Surgical removal, or Crohn's disease of the terminal ileum, may result in B_{12} deficiency but not PA. Treatment is with three-monthly injections of B_{12} in most cases. Erythropoietin is irrelevant. The Schilling test examines a patient's ability to absorb B_{12} with and without intrinsic factor and differentiates PA from other malabsorptive states that give rise to B_{12} deficiency.

232. A. T
B. T
C. T
D. F
E. T

Classically, bacterial infections result in a raised neutrophil count. Sometimes the rate of onset/severity cause temporary bone marrow arrest and agranulocytosis can develop. Myelocytes (immature granulocytes) often appear in toxic patients. If the total white blood cell (WBC) count is high this may give a blood picture similar to chronic myeloid leukaemia. Significant lymphocytosis is rare but may occur in whooping cough, for example.

233. A. F
B. F
C. T
D. F
E. T

Idiopathic thrombocytopenic purpura (ITP) is not caused by bone marrow failure; it results from excessive platelet consumption. Many, particularly adults, have a form that is truly, if temporarily, responsive to steroid therapy. Splenectomy is at best a second-line treatment. Most children, even some with prolonged thrombocytopenia, recover spontaneously. Less than 1% of children with ITP die from the disease, but the mortality is somewhat higher in adults.

234. A. T
B. F
C. T
D. T
E. F

'Reactive' thrombocytosis commonly occurs in a wide range of diseases (e.g. postoperatively in the young, in infections, vasculitis, rheumatoid arthritis) and in the young at least needs no intervention. Essential thrombocythaemia, a myeloproliferative disorder, does have a higher risk of stroke. Paradoxically, gastrointestinal tract bleeding may also occur in such patients because of abnormal platelet aggregation. A raised red cell mass associated with thrombocytosis is *typical* of polycythaemia rubra vera (PRV).

235. A. F
B. F
C. F
D. F
E. F

Haemophilia A is a sex-linked disease, the gene being on the X chromosome, caused by a low factor VIII level. Purpura are not a feature, although soft tissue and joint bleeds are common. These boys often do not present until they start walking. The bleeding time is normal. Cryoprecipitate is no longer the best form of treatment. Appropriately treated (to abolish viruses such as HIV) factor VIII concentrates should be used. Factor IX deficiency is haemophilia B (Christmas disease), also sex linked.

236. A. T
  B. T
  C. F
  D. F
  E. T

Disseminated intravascular coagulation (DIC) can be precipitated by many disorders. Severe infection and retained placenta are classic causes, as is this rare form of leukaemia. Similar microangiopathic haemolytic anaemias may be seen in haemolytic uraemic syndrome of children, but there is less consumption of clotting factors.

237. A. T
  B. F
  C. F
  D. F
  E. T

The international normalized ratio (INR) is in effect a standardized ratio of patient prothrombin time/control. Daily adjustments of the warfarin dose according to the INR will produce exaggerated 'hunting'. At least a couple of days should be left between each dose change in the early days, and longer when the patient is established. Vitamin K will disrupt anticoagulation for a long time and should be reserved for emergencies. Warfarin decreases the risk of pulmonary emboli, not stroke, in such a patient.

238. A. F
   B. F
   C. T
   D. F
   E. T

Fava bean haemolysis occurs in glucose-6-phosphate dehydrogenase (G6PD) deficiency. Haemolytic jaundice is unconjugated hyperbilirubinaemia. Autoimmune haemolysis may accompany or precede non-Hodgkin's lymphoma or other chronic lymphoproliferative disorders. In some cases splenectomy may be 'curative' since much of the red cell breakdown occurs in the spleen. Steroid treatment should be tried first. Splenectomy is a last resort.

239. A. T
   B. T
   C. T
   D. T
   E. T

Hereditary spherocytosis is an inherited haemolytic anaemia and is Coombs negative, as is glucose-6-phosphate dehydrogenase (G6PD) deficiency which, worldwide, is far more common but *not* associated with spherocytes. The red cells of this latter are sensitive to oxidizing drugs like sulphonamides. ABO haemolytic disease of the newborn, although immune mediated, is often Coombs negative.

240. A. F
   B. F
   C. F
   D. T
   E. F

Howell–Jolly bodies are nuclear remnants in red cells. They are normally nipped out as red cells traverse the spleen. They are easy to find after splenectomy. Iron (siderotic) granules in red cells are called Pappenheimer bodies, and are also a post-splenectomy feature. Heinz bodies are denatured haemoglobin and are found after oxidative damage to red cells.

241. A. T
   B. F
   C. F
   D. F
   E. F

The direct Coombs test (DCT) (or direct antiglobulin test) is
the classic way to demonstrate antibody on the surface of red
cells. It is always positive in babies with Rh haemolytic disease.
ABO blood grouping is done by directly agglutinating red
cells by the corresponding anti-A or anti-B antisera. In Coombs
positive haemolytic anaemia the strength of reaction of the
DCT is a poor indicator of the degree of haemolysis.
Transfusion of incompatible red cells may result in a positive
DCT in the recipient.

242. A. F
   B. F
   C. F
   D. F
   E. F

T lymphocytes are processed by the thymus and are long-lived.
B lymphocytes manufacture, express and may secrete
immunoglobulins. The prime line of defence against bacterial
infection is the neutrophil. Newborns have easily detectable
T cells unless they suffer from immune deficiency.

243. A. F
   B. F
   C. T
   D. T
   E. F

Neutrophils and monocytes are phagocytes. T cells reject
foreign tissue grafts. B cells express immunoglobulin
molecules on their surface – these are the specific antigen
receptors of B cells. They are one of the cell types susceptible
to infection by Epstein–Barr virus (EBV). Others include
oropharyngeal mucosa and salivary glands. T cells are
stimulated to transform by PHA.

244. A. T
B. T
C. T
D. F
E. F

Many B cell malignant proliferations can be accompanied by decreased production of normal immunoglobulins, including myeloma whose chracteristic abnormality is excess production of a single abnormal immunoglobulin (Ig) molecule. Chronic granulocytic leukaemia usually has no significant abnormality of Ig production. Chronic granulomatous disease (a rare disorder with decreased bactericidal ability of neutrophils) often has a secondary, reactive, polyclonal hypergammaglobulinaemia.

245. A. T
B. T
C. F
D. T
E. F

High dose infusion of immunoglobulin (Ig) G was first (and still is) used as replacement therapy for hypogammaglobulinaemia. It is of temporary benefit in idiopathic thrombocytopenic purpura (ITP) and in AIHA, perhaps by blocking Fc receptors of reticuloendothelial macrophages. In some patients it can provoke allergic reactions such as bronchospasm. It has no role in treating asthma or renal failure.

246. A. F
B. T
C. F
D. T
E. F

Chronic granulocytic leukaemia (CGL) is a clonal disease of haemopoiesis. The nucleated cells usually found in the largest numbers in the blood are neutrophils and their precursors, and platelets. While monocytes may also be derived from the same malignant stem cell as the granulocytes it is most unusual to find large numbers of them in the blood. Lymphocytes, for the most part, are rarely involved. The Philadelphia (Ph) chromosome is an abnormal chromosome 22 acquired, not inherited, by the clone. Constitutional trisomy 21 is of course Down's syndrome. An extra 21 in the leukaemic cells is well known in acute myeloid leukaemia.

247. A. T
B. T
C. F
D. F
E. F

While a range of viruses may possess oncogenes, many similar genes have been found in normal human DNA. Their roles are not clear but many are probably crucial in normal cell regulation. Mitochondria are complex extranuclear organelles which are not in themselves genes but do contain some DNA.

248. A. T
B. F
C. T
D. T
E. T

The breakpoint cluster region (*bcr*) of chromosome 22 fuses with the *abl* gene, translocated from chromosome 9, in the Philadelphia (Ph) translocation of chronic granulocytic leukaemia. Identical rearrangements may be found in Ph + acute leukaemias but not in polycythaemia. This rearrangement is acquired by the malignant cells and is not present in other body cells.

249. A. T
     B. T
     C. F
     D. T
     E. F

Chronic lymphatic (or lymphocytic) leukaemia (CLL) is usually a monoclonal proliferation of B lymphocytes. T cell CLL does occur but is rare, as are proliferations of NK (natural killer) cells, most of which are neither T nor B lymphocytes. Blasts are the hallmark of acute leukaemias.

250. A. T
     B. T
     C. F
     D. T
     E. F

Organomegaly is common in chronic lymphatic leukaemia (CLL). Bacterial infections are common because of the associated immune defect or marrow failure. Priapism is well described, albeit rare, in acute leukaemia and chronic granulocytic leukaemia (CGL). Central nervous system involvement is characteristic of acute lymphoblastic leukaemia and some lymphomas but rare in CLL.

251. A. F
     B. T
     C. F
     D. F
     E. T

Polycythaemia rubra vera is a primary myeloproliferative disorder with an increased red cell mass and often a raised platelet count. The expansion of red cell mass is independent of erythropoietin, whose levels are depressed or undetectable in this disease. Secondary erythrocytosis may be associated with hypoxia and renal tumours.

252. A. T
B. T
C. F
D. F
E. F

Normal adult haemoglobin (Hb A) is made up of 2 alpha and 2 beta globin chains. Hb A$_2$, a normal minor component, has 2 alpha and 2 delta globin chains. Fetal haemoglobin (Hb F) has alpha chains and gamma chains. Kappa and lambda chains are of course the light chains of the immunoglobulin molecule and have nothing to do with haemoglobin.

253. A. T
B. T
C. F
D. F
E. T

Acute lymphoblastic leukaemia (ALL) reaches its peak between the ages of 2 and 6 years. It is much less common in adults. It is much more common a cause of bone marrow failure in children than aplastic anaemia or any other infiltration of bone marrow. Cytomegalovirus infection may cause serious problems in childrem with ALL but is not known to be involved in its aetiology. Chronic lymphatic leukaemia (CLL) is treated with chlorambucil. Most ALL is a B-precursor disease, but some cases are of T cell origin.

254. A. T
B. T
C. T
D. F
E. F

Acute myeloblastic leukaemia (AML) blasts are positive while acute lymphoblastic leukaemia (ALL) blasts are negative with Sudan black staining. Nucleoli are more prominent and numerous in AML than ALL. ALL blasts usually have very little cytoplasm. The karyotype of AML cells is usually abnormal, and some types of AML have specific chromosomal abnormalities. The blasts are unable to ingest bacteria, but the more mature cells of chronic granulocytic leukaemia can do so.

255. A. T
B. F
C. T
D. F
E. T

Acute myeloblastic leukaemia, chronic granulocytic leukaemia and aplastic anaemia can all benefit from bone marrow transplants (BMT) from HLA identical siblings. Many such patients can be cured. Transplant has a very limited role in childhood ALL. Chemotherapy is the mainstay of treatment in these patients. BMT has no role in ITP (idiopathic thrombocytopenic purpura).

256. A. F
B. T
C. F
D. T
E. T

The immunological hallmark of acquired immune deficiency syndrome (AIDS) is depression of CD4 (helper) T lymphocytes. CD8 (suppressor) cells may also be depressed, especially in advanced disease. The CD4/CD8 ratio is always depressed. *Pneumocystis carinii* infection occurs in AIDS. Pneumatosis cystoides intestinalis is an irrelevant bowel condition. Intravenous drug abusers are at risk of AIDS if they share needles. There is an increased risk of lymphoma.

257. A. T
B. T
C. F
D. F
E. F

Acyclovir is important in the treatment of herpes virus infections, including herpes simplex and zoster. HVZ is not a drug! (It is the abbreviation for the virus herpes varicella-zoster.) Cytosine arabinoside and thioguanine are cytotoxic drugs with no direct role in the treatment of AIDS.

258. A. F
    B. T
    C. T
    D. T
    E. T

Myeloma is a malignant disease of plasma cells, the antibody-secreting descendants of B lymphocytes. Lytic bone lesions, pathological fractures, hypercalcaemia and renal impairment are all common. Myeloma is very rare in the young. The raised plasma viscosity (and much of the renal damage) is caused by the excessive monoclonal antibody secretion by the tumour.

259. A. F
    B. F
    C. T
    D. F
    E. F

Immunoelectrophoresis of plasma proteins is usually done to identify the light and heavy chains of a monoclonal immunoglobulin in the plasma, but other monoclonal proteins, e.g. α-fetoprotein, could also be identified in this way. It has no role in the other situations.

260. A. F
    B. F
    C. F
    D. T
    E. F

Bence-Jones protein is free monoclonal immunoglobulin light chain in the urine and is present in most cases of myeloma.

261. A. F
     B. F
     C. F
     D. F
     E. F

Heparin prevents blood coagulation. It has no effect on blood viscosity, does not lyse clots or affect capillary blood flow. It is counteracted by protamine. Vitamin K counteracts the effects of warfarin. The fibrinogen level is not affected by heparin. Heparin treatment is monitored by measurement of the activated partial thromboplastin time (APTT) or thrombin time.

262. A. T
     B. T
     C. F
     D. T
     E. T

Thymomas are associated with red cell aplasia in adults. In children transient red cell failure is usually idiopathic. Human parvovirus infection causes temporary red cell aplasia in any age group but in general only causes problems in those with a shortened red cell survivial. Congenital red cell aplasia (Diamond–Blackfan anaemia, DBA) first presents in children less than one year old, some of whom are anaemic at birth. Many with DBA are macrocytic, and most with temporary red cell aplasia develop short-lived macrocytosis as they recover. (MCV is the abbreviation for mean cell volume.)

263. A. T
     B. F
     C. T
     D. T
     E. F

Microcytic anaemia without iron deficiency is characteristic of beta thalassaemia, but patients with the trait have no particular reason for abnormally elevated ferritin levels in contrast to those with thalassaemia major. Among the red cell abnormalities, stippling of occasional cells can be striking. The haemoglobin (Hb) electrophoresis pattern is normal and will not help confirm or exclude beta thalassaemia trait.

264. A. F
     B. F
     C. T
     D. F
     E. T

Alpha thalassaemias are defects in production of the alpha chain of haemoglobin, and are associated with a relative excess of beta chains. Iron deficiency is no less common in people with alpha thalassaemia than in anyone else. While much more common in Asians it also occurs in Africans, and even in northern Europeans.

265. A. T
     B. F
     C. F
     D. F
     E. T

The fetus's haemoglobin level is substantially higher than a normal adult's: 18 g/dl is normal. Immunoglobulin (Ig) G is transferred across the placenta and is always present. IgM cannot cross the placenta and any present must have been made by the fetus. The presence of IgM should raise the possibility of an intrauterine infection of the fetus.

266. A. T
     B. F
     C. F
     D. T
     E. T

Epstein–Barr virus causes infectious mononucleosis. It is common in children, although often subclinical. The prominent 'glandular fever' syndrome is more common in adolescents who escaped childhood infection. The virus is excreted in saliva, hence the term 'kissing disease'. Splenomegaly is well described in both children and older patients. The abnormal mononuclear cells are lymphocytes not monocytes and appear to be mainly T cells, perhaps reacting against the infected B cells, pharyngeal and salivary gland cells.

267. A. T
B. T
C. F
D. T
E. T

In the UK parasites, worms in particular, and allergy account for the vast majority of cases of eosinophilia. Polyarteritis is a rare but famous cause of hypereosinophilia. Of the parasites common in the UK, *Toxocara canis* is the most likely cause of massive eosinophilia in children.

268. A. F
B. T
C. F
D. F
E. T

In patients taking warfarin, paracetamol is a safe analgesic. Aspirin should be forbidden. Barbiturates *decrease* the action of warfarin by inducing hepatic enzymes.

269. A. F
B. T
C. F
D. T
E. T

Cimetidine *enhances* the action of warfarin, as do many non-steroidal anti-inflammatory drugs. Useful lists of drugs and their effects on warfarin can be found in the *British National Formulary.*

270. A. T
B. F
C. T
D. F
E. F

Vincristine and prednisolone are included in most regimens for inducing remission in acute lymphoblastic leukaemia. Oxymethalone is an anabolic steroid with no role in treating this disease. Melphalan is used to treat myeloma or in conditioning for bone marrow transplantation. Allopurinol reduces the risk of hyperuricaemic renal damage when large numbers of tumour cells are lysed, but is not an antileukaemic drug.

271. A. T
B. T
C. F
D. T
E. T

Shingles (localized herpes varicella-zoster infection, HVZ), cytomegalovirus and disseminated herpes simplex infections can be very severe. Measles is an important, and potentially lethal, virus infection in children being treated for a variety of malignancies. Rhinovirus infection rarely causes more than a cold.

272. A. F
B. F
C. T
D. F
E. F

A CD (cluster of differentiation) antigen has been recognized by international workshops as a single antigen, of which one or more epitopes can be recognized by a range of specific monoclonal antibodies. CD antigens are given a unique number so that they may be thus identified, rather than by specifying the particular commercially available (or research institute derived) monoclonal antibody. The combinations of CD antigens on cell surfaces give indications of the tissue of origin, lineage or level of differentiation of cells from a variety of tissues.

273.   A.   T
      B.   T
      C.   F
      D.   T
      E.   F

Monoclonal antibodies are produced by a single clone of genetically identical B/plasma cells. Each antibody molecule is therefore identical to the others made by that clone. They may occur naturally, e.g. in myeloma, or be produced in the laboratory by cell culture or in experimental animals. They are not artificially synthesized. Some are of value in treatment and are administered to patients. Most are of value as laboratory reagents for identifying specific antigens, e.g. cell surface or CD antigens, or oncogene products.

274.   A.   F
      B.   T
      C.   F
      D.   F
      E.   T

Serum ferritin may be elevated into or above the normal range by other conditions, even in iron-deficient patients. Pitted nails are a feature of psoriasis. One-day-old infants are not iron deficient, whatever the iron status of the mother. Iron deficiency may decrease the response to B_{12} or folate. Treatment of megaloblastic anaemia often reveals underlying iron deficiency.

275.   A.   T
      B.   T
      C.   F
      D.   T
      E.   F

There is a rise in the mean cell volume (MCV) of maternal red cells. The haemoglobin usually falls, despite a rise in red cell mass, as a result of expansion of the plasma volume. Iron deficiency is common. Its typical microcytosis may be masked by the normal tendency for the MCV to rise or by concomitant folate deficiency.

276. A. F
      B. T
      C. T
      D. F
      E. T

Penicillin may cause allergic reactions or autoimmune haemolytic anaemia, but not aplastic anaemia. Chloramphenicol remains one of the most common iatrogenic causes of aplasia in countries where it is freely available 'over the counter'. Vincristine is useful in the treatment of a range of lymphoid malignancies but its major dose-limiting toxicity is neuropathy. It has almost no detectable effect on red cell, granulocyte or platelet production.

277. A. T
      B. T
      C. F
      D. F
      E. F

A wide range of drugs may cause haemolysis. Penicillins and cephalosporins and methyldopa are amongst those that cause immune haemolysis. Quinine and sulphonamides cause oxidative damage. Paracetamol does not cause haemolysis.

278. A. T
      B. T
      C. T
      D. T
      E. F

Splenectomy, for whatever reason, results in increased susceptibility to serious infection with pneumococcus and *Haemophilus influenzae*. Immunization against some strains is available. Lifelong penicillin prophylaxis may also reduce the risk of pneumococcal infection. Virus infections are not affected. All patients will have some rise, at least, in the platelet count after splenectomy. One of the spleen's normal roles is to remove senescent red cells. Increased fragmented or damaged red cells is common after splenectomy.

279. A. T
    B. T
    C. T
    D. T
    E. T

Fever, weight loss and night sweats are the classic 'B' symptoms of Hodgkin's disease and correlate with worse outlook.
Itching, also a prominent symptom in primary biliary cirrhosis and polycythaemia rubra vera, may be prominent. Among the peripheral blood abnormalities, microcytic anaemia (not caused by iron deficiency), eosinophilia, lymphopenia and thrombocytosis are all well described, but normocytic rather than microcytic anaemia is more common.

280. A. F
    B. F
    C. F
    D. T
    E. F

Both African and non-African Burkitt's lymphomas are tumours of B cell origin. The African form is associated with Epstein–Barr virus. The jaw is a common site of the tumour in Africans. In non-African Burkitt's, the central nervous system (CNS) and bone marrow often become involved.
Chlorambucil, useful in chronic lymphatic leukaemia, has no impact. Aggressive combination chemotherapy is required for non-African Burkitt's.

281. A. T
    B. F
    C. T
    D. T
    E. F

The management of PRV may involve venesection and/or busulphan or hydroxy urea and/or radioactive phosphorus. Hyperbaric oxygen and methotrexate have no role.

282. A. T
B. F
C. T
D. T
E. F

Severe neutropenia results in susceptibility to bacterial and fungal infections but not viral infections. *Pneumocystis carinii* is a protozoan which infects those with abnormal immune systems, whatever their neutrophil count; it is a major problem in AIDS and a recognized problem in some marrow transplant recipients and those undergoing immunosuppressive chemotherapy.

283. A. F
B. F
C. T
D. F
E. F

While all of these (and other technical errors too) may occur, clerical errors in requesting blood, completing patient details, labelling bottles, obtaining samples and recording the results of laboratory tests are the most common, simplest and most effective methods of causing a severe, and perhaps fatal, blood transfusion 'accident'.

284. A. T
B. T
C. F
D. F
E. F

The increased rate of red cell destruction leads to elevated unconjugated bilirubin levels. The compensating increase in red cell production is manifest by a raised reticulocyte count. Bilirubinuria is caused by *conjugated* hyperbilirubinaemia which occurs in obstructive jaundice and, to a degree, in hepatitis. Reticulin is young collagen in the bone marrow and is unaffected by haemolysis. Reticulin has nothing to do with reticulocytes.

285. A. F
     B. T
     C. F
     D. T
     E. F

Free haemoglobin in the urine means intravascular haemolysis whether mechanical, e.g. with artificial heart valves, or in 'march' haemoglobinuria, or even in some severe autoimmune haemolytic states. Urinary tract infections, stones, renal tract tumours and glomerulonephritis cause haematuria.

286. A. T
     B. T
     C. F
     D. F
     E. T

The genes that code for factors VIII and IX are on the X chromosome. The others are on autosomes (i.e. not sex chromosomes).

287. A. T
     B. T
     C. T
     D. T
     E. T

The telangiectases may be present in many organs. All can bleed. All these findings are well recognized in HHT. Arteriovenous malformations/shunts in the lungs can be large enough to lead to heart failure. The microcytosis is caused by iron deficiency.

288. A. F
B. F
C. T
D. F
E. F

The only important, common cause of large numbers of spider naevi is liver disease. They should not be mistaken for purpura, bruises or telangiectases.

289. A. T
B. F
C. F
D. T
E. F

Teardrop poikilocytes, red cells shaped like a teardrop on the blood film, are classically associated with myelofibrosis, and to a lesser degree with megaloblastosis. The characteristic poikilocyte of iron deficiency is the 'pencil' cell. Renal failure may be associated with 'burr' cells.

290. A. T
B. T
C. F
D. T
E. F

Fever and neutrophils in the cerebrospinal fluid (CSF) are exceptionally rarely caused by central nervous system (CNS) leukaemia. If found, they should suggest infective rather than malignant meningitis.

291. A. T
   B. T
   C. F
   D. T
   E. F

A high protein level may both discolour the cerebrospinal fluid (CSF) and give it an opalescent quality. White cells of any sort, and red cells, may cause cloudy CSF at counts as low as 100 cells/μl, but one would need to try very hard to get enough glove powder granules into the bottle to create this effect. Glucose concentrations are irrelevant.

292. A. T
   B. F
   C. F
   D. F
   E. T

Normal cerebrospinal fluid (CSF) contains up to 4–5 white cells/μl. It is often difficult to find any white cells in normal CSF. Some viral meningitides, e.g. mumps, may have surprisingly high numbers of neutrophils in the CSF. The presence of nucleated red cells and myelocytes suggests that the needle entered a vertebra and sampled the bone marrow. Xanthochromia, yellow discoloration, suggests a previous bleed, such as a subarachnoid haemorrhage.

293. A. F
   B. T
   C. F
   D. F
   E. F

Ethylenediamine tetra-acetic acid (EDTA) is the anticoagulant for blood counts. Citrate may be preferable for the very rare patients whose platelets aggregate in EDTA. Citrate is the anticoagulant of choice for clotting studies. Heparin is useful for samples whose white cells are to undergo surface marker or cell culture studies. Blood clots without an anticoagulant and is unsuitable for blood counts, but is useful for the transfusion laboratory. Dextran is not an anticoagulant.

294. A. F
 B. F
 C. T
 D. F
 E. F

The end-point is usually agglutination of red cells. Some anti-A and anti-B antisera can lyse target red cells but such antisera are not used as blood grouping agents. Rouleaux are caused by other proteins inducing the red cells to form 'stacks of coins'. This is not an immune-based phenomenon. Clotting results from the formation of fibrin and is irrelevant.

295. A. F
 B. T
 C. T
 D. F
 E. F

D-dimers are breakdown products of fibrin and are raised in a range of microangiopathic haemolytic anaemias and consumptive coagulopathies, although rather more rarely in haemolytic uraemic syndrome of children. They may often be found in those with a resolving deep vein thrombosis or after a pulmonary embolus.

296. A. T
 B. T
 C. T
 D. F
 E. T

Fanconi's anaemia is a form of inherited marrow failure. Most myelodysplastic syndromes have pancytopenia. While acute leukaemias usually have circulating blasts, they may present simply as bone marrow failure. The lymphocyte count is always raised, by definition, in chronic lymphocytic leukaemia.

297. A. F
   B. F
   C. T
   D. F
   E. F

Shock, perhaps death, is likely. There has been insufficient time for blood volume reconstitution and haemodilution to take place. As this happens, normochromic normocytic anaemia will develop. Chronic bleeding will lead to microcytic anaemia, low ferritin and increased iron-binding capacity.

298. A. T
   B. F
   C. F
   D. T
   E. T

Patients who require regular blood transfusions almost inevitably develop haemosiderosis. Peptic ulceration leads to iron deficiency eventually.

299. A. T
   B. T
   C. F
   D. T
   E. T

Chronic renal failure and polycythaemia rubra vera are the two conditions classically associated with low or absent erythropoietin levels, but only in renal failure does one want to increase the haemoglobin level! Erythropoietin has revolutionized the quality of life of many with chronic renal failure. Congenital red cell aplasia is associated with some of the highest recorded plasma erythropoietin levels of any disease.

300. A. T
B. T
C. F
D. F
E. T

Sideroblasts are normal nucleated red cells containing up to three or four granules of iron, detected by the Prussian blue staining reaction. In the bone marrow they are decreased or absent in iron deficiency. Pathological and ring sideroblasts can be found in acute leukaemias, myelodysplastic syndromes and sideroblastic anaemias and, in haemopoietic malignancies, may well belong to the malignant or premalignant clone.